THE FACTS ABOUT DIABETES

DID YOU KNOW:

- 6.5 million Americans have been diagnosed with diabetes as of 1987. Diabetes afflicts 3% of all North American adults.

- Doctors diagnose 500,000 new cases of diabetes each year.

- For every case diagnosed, another remains undiagnosed—thus *the total number of Americans with diabetes is probably well over 12 million.*

- The economic toll taken by diabetes is estimated at $20.4 billion each year.

The good news about diabetes is that you *can* take control and live a normal, healthy life with the help of the facts, information, and sources you'll find in . . .

WHAT YOU CAN DO ABOUT DIABETES

THE DELL MEDICAL LIBRARY

THE DELL MEDICAL LIBRARY

What You Can Do About
DIABETES

Norra Tannenhaus

Foreword by Steven V. Edelman, M.D.

A LYNN SONBERG BOOK

Medical research about diabetes is ongoing and subject to interpretation. Although every effort has been made to include the most up-to-date and accurate information in this book, there can be no guarantee that what we know about diabetes today won't change with time. Furthermore, diabetes sometimes displays symptoms that may appear to be related to other ailments. The reader should bear in mind that this book is not for the purpose of self-diagnosis or self-treatment; he or she should consult appropriate medical professionals regarding all medical problems and before undertaking any major dietary changes.

Published by
Dell Publishing
a division of
Bantam Doubleday Dell Publishing Group, Inc.
1540 Broadway
New York, New York 10036

For information address: Lynn Sonberg Book Services,
166 East 56 Street, New York, NY 10022

The trademark Dell® is registered in the U.S. Patent and Trademark Office.

ISBN: 0-440-20640-5
Published by arrangement with Lynn Sonberg Book Services

Printed in the United States of Americ..
Published simultaneously in Canada

June 1991

10 9 8

OPM

CONTENTS

FOREWORD

Speaking both as a diabetic and a physician who treats diabetics, I know that effective diabetes management requires motivation. It takes a motivated person to educate him- or herself about diabetes, and to follow the proper therapy program. Ideally, this program should be developed by a diabetes team consisting of a diabetologist, a nurse-educator who specializes in diabetes, a dietitian who is knowledgeable about the diabetic diet, and a podiatrist experienced in the field of diabetic foot care. The most important member of the team, however, is you, the patient, for you must take the ultimate responsibility for the day-to-day management of your condition.

The most powerful message in this book is that diabetes does not invariably lead to disability and an early death. I feel that all diabetics should use their disease as an opportunity to take extra good care of themselves, so that they may live healthier and even longer than if they'd never been diagnosed with diabetes. This book will give you a good foundation in the basics of diabetes management. It does *not* contain the rigid rules and regulations so often found in earlier books on the subject, and this is appropriate, for every diabetic is different and no two patients should be treated the same way. Thus, a strong foundation of knowledge plus practical experience are necessary for you to be able to control your diabetes and still live your life to the fullest.

Perhaps the best way for you to maintain your motivation is to experience the benefits that result when you take responsibility for your care. This, in turn, can happen only if you're knowledgeable and able to help your health-care team develop a program best suited to your needs. As long as you keep this in mind, you can pursue any goal you want —to be a doctor or a rock star; to raise a family or travel the world. This is truly the good news about diabetes.

STEVEN V. EDELMAN, M.D.
Clinical Assistant Professor
Oregon Health Sciences Center
Portland, Oregon

INTRODUCTION

Diabetes is one of the commonest conditions in America today. Consider these facts:

- Six and a half million Americans have been diagnosed with diabetes as of 1987.

- Doctors diagnose five hundred thousand new cases every year.

- For every case diagnosed, another remains undiagnosed —thus *the total number of Americans with diabetes is probably well over twelve million.*

- Diabetes afflicts three percent of all North American adults: one percent of all young adults; six percent of all middle-aged adults; and as many as ten percent of all elderly adults. Some fifteen percent of all nursing-home residents have some form of diabetes.

- The economic toll taken by diabetes is estimated at $20.4 billion each year.

Yet, despite its enormous impact, diabetes is widely mis-understood, and too frequently undetected. The American Diabetes Association (ADA) recently surveyed a thousand people and found that while eighty-five percent of those people had been tested for high blood pressure within the last three years, only half—fifty percent—had been tested for diabetes. What's more, while one of every two people asked could quote their blood-pressure level, only one of every ten knew their blood-sugar level—and yet your blood sugar remains the best available indication of the presence of diabetes.

Associated with much of the confusion surrounding dia-betes are horror stories about the complications that diabe-tes can bring—blindness, amputation, heart disease, an early death. Twenty-five percent of those in the ADA sur-vey believed that decreasing sugar intake would lower the risk of developing the disease. And many people still cling to the myth that diabetes destroys the chances for a "nor-mal" life, one that includes a good job, hobbies and vaca-tions, favorite foods, even marriage and children.

All too often diabetics themselves retain these ancient beliefs. What's even more discouraging, many doctors cling to them as well. The result: needless fear, confusion, and shame.

"I never told any of my boyfriends that I had diabetes," said Susan, who was diagnosed at age twelve. "I was afraid they'd think I was damaged in some way, or weird, or strange. If I went out on a date, I'd just try to predict our meals and activities as best I could and time my insulin accordingly. Sometimes I'd have to excuse myself and run to the nearest bathroom and shoot up." She added sadly, "More often than not I'd just turn down the invitation. It was too much trouble."

Robert learned he was diabetic three days before his twentieth birthday. "When I told my grandmother, she said, 'It's because of all that junk you love to eat. I always told your mother not to let you drink so many Cokes.' Well, that made me feel terrible—like I had brought the disease on myself in some way."

Sally, who's had a weight problem all her life, developed diabetes when she was forty-eight. "All my doctor told me was that my blood sugar was a little high, but that if I lost the weight I'd be fine. But I've already tried every diet in the world and I always gain the weight back. How can I lose weight and keep it off? How do I know which diets are healthy for me? And besides, how do I know that if I do lose the weight that everything will be okay? I have lots of questions, and he just doesn't seem to want to answer them."

The real tragedy behind these stories is that they could have been avoided so easily. Medical knowledge about the causes and treatment of diabetes has skyrocketed in the last decade. There's lots of good news about diabetes.

THE GOOD NEWS ABOUT DIABETES

Today, most diabetics can lead perfectly normal lives. They can pursue any career they wish, participate in sports, have children, eat normally—in short, with the right information and guidance, and a commitment to proper self-care, they can do anything they want. In this book you'll learn how to find health professionals who will give you the time and the guidance you need. What's more, you'll learn why it's so important to take charge of your care through proper diet, exercise, medication, and scrupulous attention to blood-glucose levels.

Doctors now know that a high-sugar diet does not cause diabetes. While many cases of diabetes are associated with obesity, sugar is not the culprit—too many calories are, regardless of the food in which they're consumed.

Doctors also believe that with proper management, most diabetics can delay, if not completely avoid, the complications associated with the disease, such as eye problems, infections, and the nerve damage known as neuropathy. In those cases where complications do occur, new treatments often prevent them from becoming too severe.

In addition, thanks to the strides made in diabetes treatment in general and the care of pregnant diabetics in particular, people with diabetes can now marry and have children almost as easily as anyone else. The idea that women with diabetes cannot bear children dates from the nineteen thirties, when nearly fifty percent of the babies born to these women died. But that figure has declined steadily over the years to two to four percent today. If you're a diabetic woman who's thinking of having children, this book will show you how to maximize your chances for a safe and healthy pregnancy.

Thus the good news about diabetes is simply this: Diabetics can lead normal lives, with a few adjustments in routine and careful planning and management. Today most diabetics remain healthy and active even after having the disease for twenty, thirty, even fifty years. In fact, many doctors find that their diabetic patients take better care of themselves than they would have if they hadn't developed the disease—and may even live longer than if they had never had diabetes in the first place!

TAKING CONTROL

The quality of your life as a diabetic depends largely on the amount of time and effort you're willing to devote to monitoring and controlling the level of your blood sugar. Self-care isn't merely helpful—it's *essential* to the successful control of your diabetes. And the secret to effective self-care is education. You owe it to yourself to learn all you can about your condition, from support groups, health professionals, radio and television programs, and books like this one. According to some studies people newly diagnosed with diabetes receive a minimum of twelve hours of individual instruction from doctors, dietitians, and other experts; some authorities think patients need as many as forty hours to learn all the aspects of diet, blood-glucose control, and appropriate medical care—along with regular updates and reevaluation.

WHY YOU NEED THIS BOOK

What You Can Do About Diabetes uses three basic elements to enhance your education. First, it provides *facts* about diabetes and explodes the myths that may be lingering in your mind or the minds of your loved ones. Second, it contains *explanations* of the metabolic processes involved in diabetes and its complications, thus clarifying the reasons why certain things go wrong. Finally, this book will provide *sources of more information.*

In Chapter One you'll learn about normal metabolism and how diabetes changes it; you'll also learn about the two major types of diabetes and who gets each type. Chapter

Two discusses diagnosis and offers suggestions for finding a doctor. Chapter Three covers the role of insulin in the treatment of diabetes, including the different kinds of insulin, the most popular dosing regimens, and the importance of tailoring insulin administration to fluctuations in blood glucose. In addition there's a discussion of drugs called oral hypoglycemics, which some people use instead of insulin.

Chapter Four is about diet, which many experts believe is the cornerstone of successful diabetic control. In addition to explaining what exchange lists are and why they're so important, this chapter contains the latest recommendations of the American Diabetes Association and offers suggestions for planning meals and snacks, and for handling emergencies. In this chapter you'll also learn about the role of exercise in the management of diabetes: it helps control blood sugar, it keeps your weight down, and it may prevent the development of heart disease, for which diabetics are at particular risk. This chapter shows you that having diabetes does require some alterations in your daily routine; Chapter Five shows you how two hypothetical patients meet the challenges of a typical day.

Chapter Six addresses the issue of complications: what they are, how they can be avoided, and how to treat them if they do occur. In addition there's a section on dental care for the diabetic and the special precautions diabetics must use when caring for their teeth.

People with special needs are the subject of Chapter Seven, which discusses the pregnant diabetic, diabetes in very young children and adolescents, and diabetes in the elderly. And in Chapter Eight you'll learn where to go for more information and support. This chapter has information about organizations that will serve as reliable sources of both long after you've finished this book.

* * *

By now you may have realized that this book emphasizes two things: good self-care, and the importance of up-to-date information. You can't have one without the other. So remember: your education doesn't end with this book. It only begins here.

WHAT IS DIABETES?

Diabetes is caused by a lack or malfunction of a hormone called insulin. Insulin acts with other hormones to regulate the body's nutrient metabolism, ensuring your tissues and cells a steady stream of fuel even when you haven't eaten for several hours—or even for several days. After a meal insulin helps the body use the incoming nutrients as efficiently as possible while storing the fuel it doesn't need until the next lean period. Thus insulin and a few other hormones enable your body to maintain the blood's level of certain nutrients, most notably glucose (blood sugar), within certain limits, so that they don't rise too high after a meal or fall too low in between.

HOW YOUR BODY USES FUEL

For a clearer understanding of the symptoms and complications of diabetes, it's important to know how insulin works in a nondiabetic individual.

Imagine that it's seven o'clock in the evening and you've just finished dinner: chicken, mashed potatoes, mixed vegetables, and chocolate pudding. Along with vitamins, minerals, fiber, and water, this meal contains three elements that the body can use as energy, or fuel: carbohydrate, protein, and fat. Some of this material will be used as fuel immediately; some of it will be stored as an energy reserve; and some of the protein will be used to rebuild worn-out tissues and replenish the body's supply of enzymes and other important chemicals. At least three hormones orchestrate this process of utilizing incoming nutrients, but this discussion will emphasize one: insulin.

When you eat something, it's first digested into simpler components to allow for easy absorption into the bloodstream. The body breaks starch down into simple sugar and protein into amino acids; fat, a more complex molecule, is handled in a slightly different way. (For a more detailed look at digestion please see Chapter Four.)

A variety of organs and glands can sense the presence of protein and sugar (glucose) in the blood and adjust their function accordingly. One of these glands is called the pancreas, which is equipped with special cells that respond to a rise or fall in blood levels of sugar or amino acids by releasing or inhibiting the release of certain hormones. When blood sugar and amino acid levels are high, one set of cells, called beta cells, responds by releasing insulin.

Insulin allows glucose and amino acids to enter muscle, fat cells, and other tissue so these nutrients can be used as fuel immediately or stored for future needs. In fat tissue insulin promotes the chemical reactions that convert excess glucose into fat; it also helps fat cells extract and store fat you've absorbed from your meal. Thus insulin promotes storage and utilization of nutrients, and for this reason scientists refer to it as a storage hormone.

Now imagine that it's seven o'clock in the morning and

you've just woken up. You've had nothing to eat since you
finished dinner at seven o'clock the night before, so you've
undergone a twelve-hour fast. Nevertheless you have the
energy to turn off your alarm, get out of bed, get dressed,
and perform all the other activities necessary to start the
day. Maybe you're not even hungry, or you're running late
—maybe you won't eat anything until lunchtime, thus pro-
longing your fast even more. Yet you manage to get
through the morning. Here again your hormones play a
role.

As more and more time elapses since your last meal,
blood-nutrient levels decline. The pancreas detects this
change and releases less insulin. Instead it secretes more
of a hormone called glucagon, whose action is essentially
the reverse of insulin: it promotes the breakdown of stored
fat and carbohydrate to ensure a steady supply of fuel to
the cells, which helps keep you going until you have a
chance to eat and replenish your fuel reserves.

The nondiabetic pancreas monitors blood sugar on a minute-by-minute basis, responding instantly to the slightest
fluctuations with adjustments in the quantities of insulin,
glucagon, and other hormones it puts out. Normally these
hormone secretions never completely stop. Instead they
act together to keep blood sugar levels within strict limits.

METABOLISM IN THE
DIABETIC PATIENT

When you have diabetes, either your pancreas stops pro-
ducing insulin or your tissues stop responding to the insulin
it does produce. When this happens, glucose can no longer

enter many organs and accumulates in the blood, leading to the hallmark of diabetes: hyperglycemia, or high blood sugar. How high can the blood sugar go? A nondiabetic's sugar usually hovers around 115 milligrams per deciliter of blood, or 115 mg/dl.* Sometimes, after a high-carbohydrate meal, it may reach 160 to 180 mg/dl. In untreated diabetes, blood sugar levels may climb to 300 and, in very severe cases, as high as 1,000 mg/dl.

These simple changes—the lack of, or defect in, insulin production, and the subsequent buildup of blood glucose—are what ultimately lead to the symptoms and complications associated with diabetes. Without insulin your body can no longer convert nutrients into the energy it needs to run properly, so it responds with metabolic changes similar to those it would make if you were starving, such as breaking down skeletal and even heart muscle in an effort to obtain fuel. What's more, the body now lacks the precise metabolic control it had when insulin could interact with other hormones, causing subtle defects in organ function that exacerbate the hyperglycemia. In addition, without insulin to balance the picture, the activity of other hormones changes. This contributes even more to the diabetic's woes.

High levels of glucose in the blood affect the function of the nerves, eyes, kidneys, heart, blood vessels, and feet. Normally, when the kidneys filter waste products from the blood, they leave the glucose to circulate back through your system. But the excessive glucose levels that occur in diabetes overwhelm the kidneys, which allow some of that sugar to escape into the urine, along with extra water needed to process the urine properly. The result: sugar in

* A milligram is one thousandth of a gram, which is roughly equal to one thirtieth of an ounce. A deciliter is roughly equal to one tenth of a quart.

the urine, too frequent urination, and possible mineral imbalances and dehydration, leading to an almost unquenchable thirst.

Diabetes also affects the metabolism of fat. Because many of your tissues are starved for fuel, they'll start burning fat instead of glucose. During this process the cells produce waste products called ketones or ketone bodies, which some organs may use as an emergency form of fuel. However, these ketone bodies distort the blood's acid-base balance and lead to a condition called diabetic ketoacidosis, or DKA. If allowed to go untreated, DKA can lead to a coma, and ultimately death.

WHAT CAUSES DIABETES?

Experts now agree that diabetes may result from a variety of causes. In rare cases diseases such as cancer of the pancreas or certain hormonal disorders may lead to diabetes, as might anything that damages the pancreas, such as certain drugs or prolonged alcohol abuse.

But in most cases the causes of diabetes remain a mystery. The vast majority of diabetic patients are classified as one of two types. Doctors have some theories on how and why these types of diabetes occur, but so far there's no conclusive proof.

Type I Diabetes

Type I diabetes, also called juvenile-onset diabetes (JOD) or insulin-dependent diabetes mellitus (IDDM), accounts for about ten percent of all the cases of diabetes in the United States. This form of diabetes usually occurs in people under twenty years old, and it's been estimated that one in every seven hundred American schoolchildren is diabetic. Each year Type I diabetes strikes another ten thousand to thirteen thousand children between the ages of five and sixteen—approximately a thousand children every month. The most vulnerable ages seem to be around eight, twelve, and adolescence, all of which are periods of growth spurts and changes in hormonal activity. In all about five hundred thousand American children and young adults currently have Type I diabetes. But this disease does not exclude grown-ups. About fifteen to twenty percent of the people with Type I diabetes are adults at the time they are diagnosed.

In Type I diabetes the pancreas suddenly loses its ability to secrete or manufacture insulin. Thus people with this form of the disease must take insulin shots for the rest of their lives. No one is certain why this disease occurs, but most experts now believe that a virus may attack the pancreas's insulin-producing beta cells. In response the immune system develops antibodies that destroy those cells as if they themselves were the invaders. In fact some investigators have found specific antibodies, called islet-cell antibodies because the beta cells occur in clusters called the islets of Langerhans, in as many as ninety percent of children who later develop diabetes.

Type II Diabetes

Type II diabetes, also referred to as maturity-onset diabetes (MOD) or noninsulin-dependent diabetes mellitus (NIDDM), accounts for about ninety percent of the cases of diabetes seen in North America. Approximately six million American adults are currently known to have Type II diabetes, and there's probably an equal number of people who haven't been diagnosed yet. As with Type I diabetes, however, Type II is not exclusive to one age group: about five percent of the people who develop this form of diabetes are under twenty years old. Many Type II patients have a parent or close relative who also has the disease.

In the vast majority of cases—estimates run from sixty to eighty-five percent—Type II diabetes is associated with obesity. In fact obesity is probably the strongest risk factor for developing Type II diabetes. For every twenty percent of excess body weight your chances of getting Type II diabetes double. Your chances also rise the longer you have the excess weight. By the same token all but a relatively few cases of Type II diabetes can be controlled through weight loss and sensible exercise. On the other hand not everyone with Type II diabetes is obese.

Unlike the Type I patient the Type II diabetic does not completely lose his or her ability to secrete or manufacture insulin. In some cases insulin-producing capacity declines; in others the pancreas can still make enough insulin but it can no longer monitor blood-glucose levels effectively. Sometimes the insulin that's produced is faulty in some way, so the tissues do not respond, and sometimes the tissues themselves change, again with the result that they don't respond to the insulin in the blood. In most cases it's probably a combination of factors.

As with Type I diabetes, no one knows what causes Type II. The condition in which insulin is present in the blood but the tissues do not respond is called insulin resistance, and is thought to be related to the number of insulin receptors on cell surfaces. As the name implies, insulin receptors are areas on the cell membrane that respond to circulating insulin by allowing glucose or amino acids to enter the cell. The insulin receptors function as "locks," with insulin itself being the "key" that opens the locks and allows glucose to enter the cells. Many experts believe that, for some reason, the insulin receptors in people with Type II diabetes are fewer, or less efficient. Muscle cells seem to be particularly prone to developing insulin resistance. Along with losing weight, regular exercise seems to diminish insulin resistance, perhaps by increasing the number of insulin receptors on muscle-cell surfaces.

TYPE I *VERSUS* TYPE II

Type I and Type II diabetes are two different disorders with the same end result. In Type I diabetes the pancreas completely loses its ability to secrete insulin. Type II most likely combines diminished or defective insulin secretion with insulin resistance. Both types lead to hyperglycemia and the inability of cells to use the energy nutrients properly. Both types also require sound medical advice and scrupulous self-care. In the next chapter you'll learn how diabetes is diagnosed—and how to find the best available help.

DIAGNOSING DIABETES

"I just started feeling tired all the time. My legs felt really heavy, and I'd feel nauseous and irritable," said Jim, a high-school senior who's had diabetes since he was nine. "Finally my parents took me to the doctor, and after running some tests he diagnosed my diabetes."

"I developed this sore on my foot about three months ago that just wouldn't go away," recalls Erica, who, at age fifty, has had a weight problem most of her life. "It didn't hurt or anything—I just looked down one night and it was there. My podiatrist couldn't find anything wrong with me, so he told me to go to the doctor for some blood sugar tests. Sure enough, I had diabetes."

Diabetes has several classic symptoms, but, as in Jim's case, it may also appear in unexpected ways. Many patients, like Erica, don't realize they have diabetes until it's discovered as part of a routine checkup, or during treatment for something else, like Erica's foot ulcer. That's why it's important to know if you run a higher-than-average risk of developing diabetes and, if you do, to get regular checkups and blood sugar tests.

The three major risk factors for diabetes are age, heredity, and obesity. The older you are, the greater your risk of being diabetic; according to some studies your chances of becoming diabetic double with every ten years of increasing age. A significant portion of all nursing-home residents have the disease. Your risk is also greater if diabetes runs in your family, particularly if it's occurred in a parent or sibling. If both your parents have diabetes, your chances of getting it are about sixty percent. With one diabetic parent you stand a three percent chance of developing diabetes between the ages of forty and fifty-nine, a ten percent chance after age sixty.

Finally, obesity—the condition of being twenty percent or more above ideal body weight—sharply raises your risk of diabetes. It's been estimated that every twenty percent of excess weight doubles your risk of developing the condition. Thus it's a good idea to maintain ideal body weight through a sensible diet and exercise (please see Chapter Four), especially if you have other risk factors for the disease.

SYMPTOMS OF DIABETES

While some cases present themselves in unconventional ways, diabetes does have some unmistakable symptoms. These include:

- Excessive urination and thirst, sometimes leading to dehydration

- Rapid weight loss, often despite constant hunger and excessive food intake

- A high level of blood glucose

- Feelings of weakness or fatigue

- Blurred vision

- Problems with sexual organs or sexual performance, including:

    —recurring vaginal or urinary tract infections, due to high levels of sugar in the blood and body tissues, which allow foreign organisms to proliferate

    —itching in the anal or genital areas, due possibly to skin infections in those areas or to overall skin dryness resulting from dehydration

    —menstrual irregularities, possibly because of hormonal changes

    —impotence and other sexual problems in men, thought to arise for a variety of reasons

Other symptoms:

- Numbness or tingling of the limbs

- A heavy feeling in the legs

- Dizziness

- Slow healing of infections or wounds

- Below-average body temperature

If allowed to progress untreated, diabetes may lead to a condition known as diabetic ketoacidosis (DKA), which results when the body is forced to burn fat instead of glucose. This can alter the blood's acid-base balance and interferes with normal metabolism, particularly in the brain. DKA may ultimately cause a coma and even death. Fortunately doctors discover the vast majority of cases of diabetes before the symptoms become severe.

The symptoms of Type I and Type II diabetes are usually similar, but there are differences in the way the two types occur. Type II diabetes occurs gradually, often over a period of years. Sometimes there are no symptoms at all until late in the disease.

Type I, on the other hand, strikes abruptly. Its victims are young and generally thin. While this form of diabetes often presents the classic symptoms mentioned earlier, in children it may also mimic the flu or gastroenteritis, with such symptoms as nausea, vomiting, and abdominal pain. Add to this the fact that, for some reason, most new cases of Type I diabetes occur between November and March, and it's not hard to see how the disease may first be misdiagnosed as some winter bug. If your child has these symptoms, see your doctor at once, particularly if the symptoms persist or if diabetes runs in your family.

MAKING THE DIAGNOSIS

To confirm a diagnosis of diabetes your doctor will measure your blood sugar before you eat breakfast, after an overnight fast of eight hours or more. In some cases the doctor may also measure your blood glucose after a meal. If your fasting blood sugar is more than 140 mg/dl, and you have other symptoms of diabetes as well, such as excessive urination or thirst, or if your postprandial (after a meal) blood sugar is greater than 200 mg/dl on two separate occasions, your doctor will diagnose diabetes.

NOW WHAT?

Most newly diagnosed diabetics require hours of instruction on topics like diet, exercise, medication, and how to handle traveling, emergencies, and sick days. They also need guidance on related subjects like eye care, foot care, dental care, pregnancy planning—the list is endless. Nor is this initial education enough. The quality of your care depends upon up-to-date assessment and evaluation, so you'll probably be visiting your doctor at least once a month, and other professionals, like a nutritionist, at least once and sometimes twice a year. In addition you owe it to yourself to remain abreast of current developments through membership in classes, support groups, and special organizations, or through subscriptions to publications.

At first all of these changes may seem overwhelming. After a while, however, you'll probably find that they've become second nature. In fact, once you've determined the best way to manage your condition, you'll undoubtedly discover that, like most diabetics, you can pursue a normal life.

Your doctor plays an important role in helping you adjust to life with diabetes. A good physician will treat not just your immediate problems; he or she can be a resource for more information and refer you to the other professionals you'll need to consult. But the quality of your care ultimately depends on you, and the best way to assure high-quality care is to find the best doctor you can.

What to Consider
When Searching for a Doctor

Your chances of finding the right doctor for you will be greatly improved if you know what you want in a doctor before you begin your search. Up-to-the-minute knowledge about treating diabetes is, of course, the main prerequisite, but if you have other health problems you may feel more comfortable with a general practitioner who can treat your other ailments and refer you to a diabetes specialist when necessary. Accessibility is also important; diabetic patients often require more of a physician's time than other patients, so you may want to find someone whose patient load isn't so heavy that he won't be able to give you the attention you need. When you visit a new doctor, you may want to ask yourself the following questions:

- Do I feel comfortable with this person?

- Are his instructions clear? Does he answer my questions patiently and thoroughly?

- Does he interact well with my family?

- Is his office staff courteous and accessible?

- Does his treatment work?

- Does he listen to me? Take my fears and questions seriously? Respect my thinking when I make a suggestion about my treatment?

- Can he refer me to other health professionals should I need further treatment?

- How up to date is his knowledge about diabetes? (You may be able to get an idea by looking at the medical journals he keeps around his office, by checking with a medical library for any books or articles he may have written, or by asking if he holds any teaching positions.)

- If this doctor is a general practitioner, does he know enough about diabetes care to realize when he should send me to a specialist?

- Are his examinations thorough? As a diabetic you should regularly have your heart, blood pressure, cholesterol, kidneys, eyes, and feet checked—not necessarily all of them at every examination, but often enough to offer a current picture of your health.

FINDING A DOCTOR

Fortunately, with all the resources currently available to diabetics, this shouldn't be difficult. The American Diabetes Association and the Juvenile Diabetes Foundation maintain chapters in most large cities; call the one nearest you and ask them to send you a list of doctors practicing in your area. If neither of these organizations has a chapter in your area, call the American Diabetes Association headquarters in Alexandria, Virginia (the 800 number is given at the end of Chapter Eight), and ask them for the nearest chapter.

Local hospitals and medical societies may also be good sources of information. Many offer classes and seminars on diabetes; attend one and chat with the people you meet there. A recommendation from a satisfied patient is often the best referral of all. If the class is taught by a physician and you like him, ask him afterward if he will take you on as a patient. Even if he can't, he may direct you to an associate.

Public libraries often contain directories of physicians in your area, or carry journals published by local medical societies. These may provide the names of some doctors in your area that you can then check out. Finally, if your community has a university or a medical school, call and ask if any of their faculty members maintain nearby offices and if they see diabetic patients.

Remember: It's a Two-Way Street

Many of the qualities you seek in the ideal physician are precisely those that physicians hope to find in the ideal patient. Just as you want a doctor who respects your opinions and communicates clearly, doctors want patients who state questions and complaints clearly and heed the doctor's advice. Give your doctor the same kind of patience and respect you desire from him, and the two of you will most likely develop a comfortable, productive relationship that may last years.

Tips for Maintaining a Good Doctor-Patient Relationship

1. Don't make snap judgments. Visit a doctor at least three or four times before you decide if he's right for you.

2. Be honest. Give accurate answers when asked about diet, medication, exercise, and whether or not you're

complying with treatment orders. Dishonest or evasive answers impair your doctor's ability to help you and ultimately diminish the quality of your care.

3. Listen to your physician as you want him to listen to you.

4. Work with your doctor to set goals for your treatment; check to make sure that your expectations are realistic; and confirm with him that you're managing your treatment properly.

5. Don't be afraid to get a second opinion or consult a specialist if you think it's necessary.

6. Make sure you know what to do when you fall ill. Ask your doctor ahead of time what to do on "sick days," such as:
   —What adjustments should I make in diet, exercise, or medication?
   —Should I check my blood glucose more often than usual?
   —At what level is blood glucose considered too high? What should I do then?
   —How much fluid should I drink, and what kind?
   —If the doctor prescribes any medication, what are its side effects and how will it interact with the diabetes medication I'm taking? Will it affect my blood sugar?
   —What kinds of over-the-counter medications may I use? (Some nonprescription drugs, like cough medicines, contain sugar and must be used with caution by a diabetic.)
   —What should I do if I don't get better?

Far from becoming too dependent on their physicians most patients find that a good doctor-patient relationship enhances their responsibility for their own care. Through good communication with their doctors and mutual respect, patients have learned to interpret their bodies' signals, stay healthy, circumvent emergencies, and avoid hospitalization. The result: fewer hospital bills, a greater feeling of responsibility for one's own care, diminished feelings of helplessness, and enhanced self-esteem.

THE GOALS OF DIABETES THERAPY

Regardless of the type of diabetes you have, your doctor's immediate therapeutic goal will be to keep your blood-sugar levels within normal limits. Type I diabetics require insulin to accomplish this; Type II patients may be controlled entirely through diet, or they may require pills known as "oral hypoglycemics." Some Type II diabetics find that diet and pills aren't enough; they require insulin for the best management of their diabetes.

The long-term goals of therapy are to minimize, delay, or entirely prevent complications and to let you live a normal life. All of this is best accomplished by achieving the immediate goal: regulating blood sugar. In the next few chapters you'll learn how drugs, diet, and exercise all help keep your blood sugar in line—and how you can make sure they work.

THE AGE OF INSULIN

Diabetes is as old as mankind; it's described in literature going back at least three thousand years. For most of that time doctors and loved ones could do little more than experiment with trial-and-error remedies and, for the most part, watch helplessly as the diabetic patient died.

All of that changed in the early nineteen twenties, when Drs. Frederick Banting and Charles Best first tried insulin in a boy dying of diabetes. He survived, becoming a witness to one of the greatest achievements in modern medicine. It's impossible to calculate the number of lives insulin has saved, worldwide, in the decades since its first clinical use, but the figure must surely reach into the millions.

Today insulin is a routine part of diabetic management, and there are several dozen brands of insulin on the market. In fact insulin has become so familiar to so many that it's easy to forget that using it involves more than just giving yourself a shot once or twice a day.

THE GOALS OF INSULIN THERAPY

In the person without diabetes the pancreas produces insulin constantly, in changing amounts that respond to minute-by-minute fluctuations in blood-glucose levels. Insulin works with other hormones produced by the pancreas and other glands to maintain the levels of glucose, fat, and amino acids in the blood, and to keep your metabolism going at an appropriate rate twenty-four hours a day.

The primary goal of current diabetes treatment is to keep metabolism and blood glucose levels as close to normal as possible, on a consistent basis. To many diabetics this means the judicious use of insulin, coordinated with their usual patterns of eating and exercising. As a diabetic you must shoulder the job your pancreas used to perform: that of monitoring blood-glucose levels and responding with appropriate changes in hormone output.

DIFFERENT KINDS OF INSULIN
AND HOW THEY WORK

Currently there are over forty types of insulin available in the United States. They're usually grouped according to the species they came from—human, pork, or beef—or the duration of their action—short, medium, and long acting.

Regular, or short-acting, insulin reaches the bloodstream and starts lowering blood sugar thirty minutes to two hours after it's injected. Its maximum activity, or peak, occurs after two to four hours, and it continues to show some activity for as long as six to eight hours after being administered. Semilente, a special type of short-acting insulin, begins acting one to two hours after injection, peaks within three to eight hours, and lasts for ten to sixteen hours.

Intermediate-acting insulins, including Lente, NPH, and PZI, begin to act within ninety minutes, peak at four to twelve hours, and last up to twenty-four hours. Finally, long-acting, or human, Ultralente insulin begins acting six to eight hours after injection, peaks anywhere from twelve to fourteen hours later, and may last for as long as twenty-four hours, providing the patient with a slow, continuous insulin release.

Pork and beef insulin are isolated from the pancreases of pigs and cattle. Pork insulin is especially similar to human insulin. People have used these products for years with good results, but there has been some danger of allergic reactions. Also, as the worldwide incidence of diabetes has grown, some experts feared that insulin demand would soon exceed supply, creating an international shortage.

Fortunately those problems seem to have been averted with the development of human insulin. Scientists use two methods to obtain human insulin: They modify animal insulin to match the chemical structure of the human hormone, or they insert human insulin-producing genes into bacteria, which then become little insulin "factories." Today the use of animal insulin is slowly being phased out: already nearly half of all insulin-requiring diabetics use human insulin, and it is prescribed for most newly diagnosed patients.

More rapidly absorbed into the blood than pork or beef insulin, human insulin is less likely to cause allergic reactions because it is purer than the other products. It acts faster, peaks earlier, and has a shorter duration than the animal insulins, and is also slightly more expensive. Nevertheless, because it's the closest thing possible to an exact replica of the insulin your own body would produce if it could, human insulin is being prescribed for more and more diabetics.

HOW OFTEN, HOW MUCH?

As recently as ten years ago you could buy insulin in four different strengths: U-20, U-40, U-80, and U-100. These numbers refer to the units of insulin in one cubic centimeter (cc) or milliliter (ml) of solution—roughly one thousandth of a quart. U-100, which has one hundred units of insulin per cc, was first introduced in 1973 and is a highly purified preparation that eliminates or minimizes many of the negative side effects formerly associated with insulin use, like insulin allergy or a deterioration of the subcutaneous fat at the injection site. Over the last few years the three lower strengths have been phased out almost entirely in the United States, making U-100 the strength most commonly found. U-40 is still occasionally used by some American patients and is the most popular insulin strength in Europe.

To achieve the best blood-glucose control, and most closely approximate the body's natural physiological state, the American Diabetes Association recommends that insulin-requiring patients use a mixture of insulins of different time duration, several times a day. This practice tries to account for the fact that different people absorb insulin at different rates, and that long-acting insulins seem to work best when combined with the shorter-acting varieties. The thought of giving yourself a shot two, three, or even four times a day may seem distasteful, but this appears to be the best way to achieve good blood-glucose control.

Ideally your insulin therapy should be tailored to your life-style, taking into account factors such as eating and exercise habits, and frequency of travel. If you've had diabetes for some time and have been using beef or pork insulin with no problems, the chances are your doctor will keep you on that regime rather than starting you on something new, unless your needs change. One widely used prescription *mixes* short- and intermediate-acting insulin and *splits* them into two or more injections per day—the "split-mixed" regimen. Or, depending on your needs, your doctor may have you vary the dose of short-acting insulin or take different kinds of insulin several times a day. One shot a day is almost never enough for the Type I patient.

Insulin Therapy in the Patient with Type I Diabetes

People with Type I diabetes produce no insulin at all, so they are absolutely dependent upon their insulin shots. Frequent reevaluation is the cornerstone of their insulin therapy; a dose that may have worked for them a year ago may not be sufficient now. The best way to determine this is through frequent checkups by a doctor, and through good self-monitoring of blood glucose (SMBG), which is described a little later in this chapter.

Insulin Therapy in the Patient
with Type II Diabetes

People with Type II diabetes may still produce some insulin, but their tissues may be resistant to it or the insulin itself may somehow be impaired. Usually these patients can regain normal glucose control by losing weight, exercising, eating properly, and not smoking. If these measures don't work, Type II patients may be given pills, known as oral hypoglycemics. A growing number of physicians, however, are prescribing insulin to their Type II patients instead. For some Type II patients insulin is essential, including patients undergoing acute physical stress, like an infection, an injury, or upcoming surgery; people who are allergic to hypoglycemic pills; and pregnant women.

There's one major drawback to insulin therapy in the Type II patient: Some doctors report that it increases appetite in some patients, leading to more eating and weight gain, which may exacerbate the diabetes. While this observation has not been confirmed by rigorous scientific studies, if you're a Type II diabetic on insulin, be alert to any changes in appetite and weight and report them to your doctor. With good nutritional management, weight gain need not be an inevitable result of your therapy.

MAKING INSULIN THERAPY
WORK FOR YOU

The whole point of insulin therapy is to maintain your blood-glucose levels as close to normal as possible. To know if you're being successful at this, the best thing to do is check your blood glucose regularly. Diabetics call this self-monitoring of blood glucose, or SMBG.

SMBG allows you to test your blood glucose at home, as often as you think necessary—some people test their blood eight times a day—and to alter your medicine, diet, and exercise if such changes are needed. Thus SMBG allows you to take control of your therapy and your life, and is recommended by the American Diabetes Association for all insulin-requiring patients.

SMBG allows you to:

- monitor blood-sugar fluctuations throughout the course of a day

- agree, with your doctor, upon target blood-sugar levels to strive for in treatment

- obtain immediate information about your blood-glucose level, letting you take action if the level seems to be approaching the limits you've set for it

Any diabetic can benefit from SMBG, but it is absolutely essential for patients who are:

- just beginning insulin therapy or changing to a new dose or regimen

- plagued by recurrent swings in blood sugar and want to find out why

- undergoing a period of physical or psychological stress

- Type I diabetics prone to frequent hypoglycemia, and who may not recognize or experience the usual warning symptoms

- using an insulin pump

- pregnant or planning pregnancy

In addition SMBG is strongly recommended for patients who:

- want good routine management of Type I diabetes
- take unusually high doses of insulin
- have kidneys that are unusually sensitive or insensitive to blood sugar levels

SMBG helps in a variety of situations. For example, blood sugar often remains elevated in Type II patients several hours after a meal. For them it's a good idea to wait until glucose levels approach normal before they eat again. SMBG can help these patients determine appropriate between-meal intervals. In other patients absorption of insulin from the injection site may vary up to twenty-five percent in the same person at different times, for reasons that remain a mystery. Through SMBG these patients can learn if they're getting the maximum benefit from their insulin.

The frequency with which you perform SMBG depends on your individual needs and treatment plan. Ideally you and your doctor should determine together certain target levels of blood sugar to aim for, using a combination of meal planning, exercise, and medication. Many doctors give their patients an algorithm, a plan of action that suggests changes to make in your meal plan, insulin dose, or exercise, based upon your blood sugar level. By freeing the patient from complete reliance upon the physician for every treatment-related decision, the algorithm allows the diabetic even more control over his or her therapy.

In a typical day a diabetic may perform SMBG four times: before each meal and at bedtime. Type II patients

Ideally, a doctor creates an algorithm after he or she has been treating the patient for a few months and has become familiar with the vicissitudes of that particular patient's case. The algorithm is different for each patient, and requires constant reevaluation.

The chart below illustrates a sample algorithm. It tells the patient how many units of insulin to take and when, depending on his blood glucose level in a prebreakfast or predinner SMBG. The algorithm may also take into account special events. For example, if the patient is planning some strenuous exercise, his doctor might advise him to take 1/2 to 1/3 the insulin dose recommended for his blood glucose level as determined by a preactivity SMBG. Exercise usually helps glucose enter the cells even if insulin isn't present, so the insulin dose must be adjusted accordingly.

Doctors may also use the algorithm to determine long-term changes in treatment. If the patient reports that he frequently needs higher doses of insulin to get his blood sugar within normal range, the physician may reasonably conclude that this person should take more insulin on a regular basis.

A SAMPLE ALGORITHM

Blood Glucose (mg/dl)	Units of Regular Insulin	
	Before Breakfast	Before Dinner
Less than 80–150	5	7
151–200	6	9
201–250	7	11
251–300	8	13
310–400	9	15

Note: On sick days, an adjustment in insulin dose is usually not necessary until blood glucose exceeds 250.

whose blood sugar is stable with diet alone or diet plus pills may require only a morning (prebreakfast) SMBG three to seven times a week, with extra readings taken once or twice a month at bedtime or before a meal. But the frequency of SMBG is highly individualized; only you and your doctor can decide what's best for you.

A Word of Caution

If you and your doctor have decided that your SMBG has to be done only before meals and at bedtime, keep in mind the fact that postprandial blood sugar levels often rise drastically. Thus, it's a good idea to take an occasional reading before and after a meal or a particular food for a clearer picture of how your blood sugar levels fluctuate. Really dramatic swings may call for a change in your meal plan, exercise routine, insulin dose, or all three.

WHAT SHOULD MY BLOOD SUGAR BE?

It's been suggested that you and your doctor set certain blood-sugar "targets" to aim for in your therapy. The question is, what should those targets be?

The American Diabetes Association considers ideal blood-sugar levels to be 80 mg/dl in the fasting state and 140 mg/dl after a meal. Acceptable levels are 70 fasting and 200 postprandial; anything less than 60 fasting or more than 240 postprandial are considered unacceptable.

It is, of course, impossible to decide upon one ideal figure as your target and then try to get your body to arrive precisely at that level, time after time. There's only so much you can do to control your blood sugar levels; after that your body takes over, and unfortunately you can't always predict how it's going to behave. Therefore, as a diabetic, you'll probably be given a target range of blood-sugar levels to strive for, with the assumption that if your readings can fall somewhere within those boundaries, your diabetes is under control. A good fasting range is 70 to 130 mg/dl; one hour after a meal the range is 100 to 180. Two hours after eating your range will probably be 80 to 150, and after that the fasting range applies once again.

ACCESSORIES AND EQUIPMENT

It's easy to become dismayed by all of this, especially if it's new to you. Insulin shots up to four times a day; planning ahead all your meals and activities; testing your blood sugar up to eight times a day—that's every three hours! And indeed, there are people who wake up in the middle of the night just to check their glucose. You're taking over for an organ whose function doctors have yet to fully understand, and although diabetes treatment has made vast strides in the last few decades, it still imposes considerable restrictions on the patient.

That's why companies are continually refining and improving the equipment that diabetics must use. The easier and less intrusive your treatment is, the more likely you'll be to adhere to it, and the more effective the treatment will be. To help with SMBG, diabetics can choose from a wide variety of glucose meters currently on the market. These devices give you instantaneous readings of your blood sugar, permitting immediate changes in control, if necessary. They're convenient (all weigh less than one pound), easy to use, and some have extra features—for example, certain models can store data for transfer to a personal computer. To use a glucose meter you put a drop of blood on a specially treated sensor or strip (special pricking devices are available), wait a few moments, rinse or wipe the blood away, and place the strip in the meter. Within thirty seconds to two minutes you'll know your blood glucose.

One step up from the blood-glucose meters are more elaborate data-management systems, which provide information about time, date, insulin type and dose, food eaten, exercise performed, and any other special circumstances that might be important, as well as your blood glucose. These minicomputers can be hooked up to a personal computer or a modem, which can transfer the data to a computer in your doctor's office. Such equipment may seem excessive to some people, but for those with special needs they help maintain tight control over blood-glucose levels, and they give physicians even more information about their patients.

In addition to such high-tech equipment there are simpler devices that help with insulin injections, offering aid to those with poor vision, for example, or to people with limited manual dexterity. There are even special insulin "pens" or "jets," for people who just can't stand giving themselves shots. Whatever your budget or needs, there's something out there for you to help make your job a little easier. Your insurance carrier may pay for much of this equipment. Most diabetes specialists or employees at diabetes clinics remain up to date about such developments; ask them for more information. In addition the American

Diabetes Association (ADA) has a monthly magazine that regularly reviews new equipment. Chapter Eight tells you how to contact the ADA.

The Insulin Pump

The insulin pump is the closest thing yet to an artificial pancreas. This electromechanical device provides a continuous infusion of insulin—the basal infusion—around the clock, while allowing the patient to deliver an extra squirt—the bolus infusion—at special times, such as just before meals. In this way the pump approximates the function of a normal pancreas. These devices are best suited for people who need more intensive insulin therapy, including:

- women who are trying to conceive—the pump is the best way to achieve good glucose control and can be used throughout pregnancy

- patients who have experienced early growth retardation or early complications of diabetes

- people with irregular schedules who may often miss or delay meals

Insulin pumps range in size; some are as small as a credit card, others as large as a videotape. Most patients wear them on their belts and detach them at certain times, as when bathing. The pump delivers the insulin through a plastic tube attached to a needle or cannula that's inserted just under the skin and taped into place. They can deliver from one tenth of one insulin unit per hour up to several units per hour, which means they allow for precise dosing to match each patient's needs.

These devices have been a boon to many, but they still have their drawbacks. Patients who use insulin pumps must monitor their blood glucose at least four times a day, and usually more. They must take the time to learn exactly how and when to adjust their food, exercise, and insulin dose to keep their blood sugar within safe limits in the face of the constant hormone infusion. For this reason it's best to have a doctor who's experienced in the use of insulin pumps, and to consult the other members of your health-care team as well. In general the successful use of an insulin pump requires a lot of motivation, a healthy shot of common sense, lots of support from your family and health-care team, and good insurance coverage: the pumps cost several thousand dollars, not including the other equipment you'll need to use them properly. It's also important to take a realistic approach. They're often likened to an artificial pancreas, but the truth is that insulin pumps do *not* cure diabetes, and they do not relieve you of the responsibility of frequent blood-glucose checks, regular visits to your doctor and other health-care practitioners, and carefully planned meals and activity. If anything, the pumps require even more vigilance than other forms of treatment.

TROUBLE SHOOTING

You're doing everything right: seeing your doctor regularly, SMBG six times a day, paying strict attention to your food, exercise, and insulin dose. Yet, despite your best efforts, your blood-glucose readings are sometimes too high or too low. What could it be? Here's a checklist of things to consider when trying to find the reason for swings in blood sugar.

1. An unexpected burst of exercise may decrease blood sugar, especially following a long period of inactivity. Did you have to run to catch the bus this morning? Climb the stairs because the elevator was broken? Park your car far away from the stores in a crowded shopping mall? While not part of a formal exercise program, these are all forms of activity that can affect your blood glucose.

2. A forgotten snack. Perhaps one of your co-workers brought in some home-baked brownies, and you had a taste. Or maybe the local supermarket was giving out free samples of food. It's a good idea to keep a food diary to help you remember such impromptu nibbles.

3. A change in the timing or composition of a meal. You were working late and couldn't get away, so you and a few other people ordered out for a pizza. There's no harm in doing this occasionally, as long as you do your SMBG and compensate for any blood-sugar changes.

4. Forgotten or underestimated stress. Stress often releases hormones that can raise your blood-sugar levels. Did you have a fight with your spouse? A crisis at work? Such temporary, day-to-day forms of stress may have more of an impact than you realize on your blood sugar.

5. The use of alcohol or certain drugs. Alcohol may not only affect your blood sugar, it can impair your ability to recognize the symptoms of hypo- or hyperglycemia. Some drugs may also impair your judgment; others may react negatively with insulin or oral hypoglycemics, with

a subsequent change in your blood sugar. If your doctor prescribes any new medication, ask him about its potential effect on the medicine you're taking now.

6. Illness or infection are forms of stress that often raise blood sugar. If your blood sugar increases and you can't explain it any other way, ask your doctor to check you for a cold, the flu, or an infection.

7. Your insulin injecting technique. If you inject insulin into your arm and then use that arm to chop vegetables, the insulin may be more rapidly absorbed and lower your blood sugar too much. Or you may have changed the depth at which you administer the injection, without realizing it. Always injecting in the same spot may lead to thickening of the skin in that area, making it more difficult to insert the needle—this is why most authorities recommend rotating the injection site. Consider asking your doctor or other diabetes professional to review with you the principles of injecting insulin.

Insulin Dos and Don'ts

1. Do keep the insulin you're currently using at room temperature, about seventy degrees Fahrenheit. Contrary to popular belief there's no need to keep your current bottle in the refrigerator; the cold temperature may make the injection needlessly painful. Do, however, store spare bottles in the refrigerator.

2. Do have at least one spare bottle of insulin always on hand, so if your pharmacy runs out of your kind, you have time to go elsewhere or order more.

3. Do take another bottle of insulin from the refrigerator when you finish your current bottle, to make it ready for your next dose.

4. Do check the expiration date on the insulin bottle before you use it.

5. Do examine the insulin before you use it. Check regular insulin for discoloration; check Lente or NPH for a frosted appearance or the development of clumps or crystals in the solution or on the bottle. Do return the unused insulin to your pharmacist if you find any of these conditions.

6. Don't shake or agitate human insulin.

7. Don't store insulin at extreme temperatures—don't place it in direct sunlight, for example, or in the freezer.

8. Don't use any insulin after its expiration date.

Glycosylated Hemoglobin Testing

SMBG illustrates day-to-day fluctuations of your blood glucose, but unless you have one of the sophisticated new devices described earlier, it's difficult to get an idea of the long-term activity of your blood glucose. That's why your doctor may sometimes perform a glycosylated hemoglobin test. This test, which is currently done only in laboratories, measures the percentage of certain kinds of hemoglobin (a component of red blood cells) to which glucose is attached. These values correlate with your total blood glucose and can be used to assess the effects of therapy over a period of six to eight weeks. Doctors consider the glycosylated hemoglobin test the most reliable assessment of blood glucose, and may use it to get an idea of your long-term blood-glucose control, or to assess the effects of a change in treatment that may have been made two months ago. Some physicians may also use this test when first evaluating a patient for diabetes.

What's Wrong with Urine Tests?

"Diabetes has run in my family for generations. I remember when my grandmother had it," says Sally, who, at fifty-five, has just been diagnosed with diabetes. "Grandma tested her urine all the time. Now they tell me urine tests are no good—I have to test my blood."

Testing the urine for glucose was once the only means available to diabetics to assess their control. It was better than nothing, but highly flawed. The results were unreliable and could be distorted by changes in fluid intake, the time since last urination, the patient's intake of vitamin C, and the technique used to perform the test. Age and kidney function also affected the test.

Current methods of SMBG have made urine glucose tests obsolete in the treatment of diabetes (although they're still better than nothing for the occasional patient who absolutely refuses to perform SMBG). But urine tests are useful for measuring something else: the presence of ketones. These may indicate the presence of diabetic ketoacidosis (DKA), a life-threatening condition that develops when the blood sugar is too high.

THE DANGER OF
GLUCOSE EXTREMES:
DKA AND HYPOGLYCEMIA

DKA

The body produces waste products called ketones when it burns fat instead of carbohydrate for fuel. This happens when you don't have enough insulin, so glucose cannot enter the cells. Instead, the sugar accumulates in the blood, and the body uses fat for energy, creating the ketones. When the blood level of ketones is too high, these substances enter the urine.

Ketones make the blood more acid in nature (hence the term *ketoacidosis*). If allowed to persist for several hours or days, DKA will affect brain function, ultimately leading to a coma and death. The symptoms of early DKA include dehydration; excessive urination or thirst; nausea and vomiting; visual problems, such as blurred vision; and abdominal pain, especially in younger diabetics.

You can test your urine for ketones in two ways. One is with the help of special tablets that change the urine's color, depending on the level of ketones present; the other is with strips treated with a chemical at one end. If ketones are present, the chemically treated end will change color when dipped into a urine specimen.

DKA occurs when you don't have enough insulin to meet your needs. This was what killed so many diabetics before the age of insulin; today it may occur following any physiological stress, like pneumonia or the flu, in patients who haven't taken enough insulin to compensate for it. It's also seen in people who forget to take their insulin, or who deliberately don't take it for some reason.

Ketones in the urine don't necessarily mean that you already have DKA, but they do indicate that it's looming on the horizon and you should seek help. Tell your doctor immediately if your urine tests positive for ketones, if your blood sugar is persistently high, if you are running a fever, or if you're vomiting or feeling nauseated.

Hypoglycemia

Too much insulin may be just as dangerous as too little. When your insulin dose exceeds your need, too much glucose enters the cells, leaving too little in the blood to go to the brain. The result: hypoglycemia, or low blood sugar. Hypoglycemia usually occurs when blood glucose dips to 50 to 60 mg/dl.

The symptoms of hypoglycemia reflect its effect on the brain. Tremors, heart palpitations, hunger, and excessive sweating are some of the early symptoms; later symptoms include drowsiness, irritability, confusion, poor coordination, loss of consciousness, and convulsions. In its early stages hypoglycemia is easily treated by having the patient consume some form of simple sugar—a nondiet soft drink, some hard candy, or one of the forms of emergency glucose currently available. The symptoms should abate in ten to fifteen minutes. Someone in the later stages of hypoglycemia may require two doses of simple carbohydrate, as well as assistance from others if judgment or coordination is impaired. An unconscious patient will need an intravenous infusion of glucose or glucagon, the hormone that raises blood sugar.

Diabetic hypoglycemia usually occurs when food intake fails to keep up with insulin or exercise levels. It's often seen in Type I diabetics who go on unsupervised low-calorie diets. Hypoglycemia may also be caused by something called the "honeymoon phase" of insulin therapy. Shortly after they start taking insulin, some newly diagnosed diabetics may experience some recovery of pancreatic function, and they start making some insulin once again. So now there's a double dose of insulin: that made by the body, and that taken by the patient. Together they cause hypoglycemia. Teenagers and young adults are the most likely candidates for a honeymoon phase, which is marked by frequent episodes of hypoglycemia. During this period the insulin dose must be decreased or, in some cases, omitted altogether.

The honeymoon phase may last as long as a year, but it is temporary. Ultimately the patient will have to resume his or her insulin injections.

A mild episode of hypoglycemia may seem fairly harmless, but it's important to avoid this condition as much as possible. Hypoglycemia may impair judgment, making it dangerous for the diabetic to operate machinery or drive a car; it may also interfere with someone's job or school performance. What's more, prolonged or repeated episodes may cause permanent damage to the nervous system, especially in young children.

One word of warning: Diabetic hypoglycemia is a genuine danger and is not to be confused with the "hypoglycemia" you may have seen mentioned in the popular press. Hypoglycemia in nondiabetics is rare and must be properly diagnosed under the right conditions by a physician.

ORAL HYPOGLYCEMICS

Some Type II diabetics do not require insulin but cannot adequately control their diabetes through diet and exercise alone. They need a group of agents known as oral hypoglycemics, which is your doctor's way of saying "pills that lower blood glucose."

The oral hypoglycemics used in the United States today are known as sulfonylureas, which are thought to act primarily by stimulating the pancreas to produce more insulin. Scientists think these products may also relieve the insulin resistance seen in Type II patients, possibly by increasing the number of insulin receptors on the cell surfaces.

Oral hypoglycemics work best on patients who develop diabetes after the age of forty, have had the disease for five years or less, and who have never taken insulin or take less than forty units per day. Sixty to seventy percent of the people who try oral hypoglycemics respond well, but some Type II patients never respond and need insulin, while others do well at first but gradually stop responding. These patients eventually require insulin.

Doctors who consider prescribing oral hypoglycemics must take into account the patient's age, weight, and general health, as well as the severity of his diabetes. It's also important for the doctor to know about any other drugs the patient is taking, since the oral hypoglycemics can interact badly with certain other agents. Possible side effects of these products include:

- severe hypoglycemia

- skin reactions, such as itching or a rash

- gastrointestinal symptoms such as nausea or vomiting

Oral hypoglycemics are not recommended for:

- pregnant women, because their effect on the developing baby isn't known

- patients who have certain infections or have undergone trauma, like an accident

- anyone who's allergic to these drugs

TIPS FOR SICK DAYS

As you've seen, catching a bug may require some important changes in your insulin schedule. Stress of any kind can raise your blood glucose, and illness is no exception. Sick days are also tricky because, if you're not feeling well, you may not want to eat, you may not be as active as usual, you may sleep through the time for your usual insulin injection, or you may take some other medication that affects your blood sugar. For all these reasons it's important to work out a sick-day game plan with your doctor and dietitian. (See Chapter Four.) The National Diabetes Advisory Board offers the following tips:

1. When you feel too sick to eat normally or stay active, call your doctor and describe in detail how you feel. *Do not delay!*

2. Continue taking your insulin when you feel sick. Do not stop taking your insulin even if you cannot eat. Your doctor may change your insulin dose.

3. Drink extra liquids if your temperature is above normal. Try to drink at least twelve eight-ounce glasses of

liquid per day if you weigh eighty pounds or more. Write down how much you drink. If you are throwing up, call your doctor right away. You may need to go to the hospital or have special medical treatment.

4. Take your temperature every morning and evening while you are sick. Use a rectal thermometer for small children or someone who is breathing through the mouth.

5. Test your urine each time you urinate. Measure its sugar and ketone content and write down both. If your urine contains ketones or two percent sugar or more, call your doctor. He may have you call him every four to six hours so he can adjust your insulin dose. He may also ask you to estimate how much urine you pass each time.

6. Weigh yourself every day while you are ill.

7. Record your rate and type of breathing every time you urinate. If you are panting, describe your breathing as "shallow." If you feel that you are breathing deeply, write "deep." If you are breathing normally, write "normal." Time your rate of breathing, using a watch. If you are taking more than twenty-four breaths per minute, or if you start having a lot of trouble breathing, call your doctor or have a family member do it for you. A change in breathing pattern is one of the signs of DKA.

8. Every time you urinate, decide how alert you feel. Write down whether you feel "sleepy" or "awake." If you feel very sleepy and cannot pay attention, have a friend or relative call the doctor *immediately*.

9. Call your doctor every day while you're sick, to tell him what you have written down regarding your temperature, weight, liquid intake, level of urinary sugar and ketones, breathing pattern, and degree of alertness. Depending on what you tell him, your doctor may adjust your insulin dose.

10. Ask a family member or friend to do these things for you if you feel too sick to do them yourself.

FOUR

DIET

The original name for this chapter was "The Diabetic Diet." But what is the "diabetic diet"? Is it a bland diet, devoid of sweets, snacks, fast foods, and other things "normal" people can have? Is it a diet whose components come from the "diabetic" or "dietetic" section in the supermarket, where the food has been formulated to taste foul and prevent instant death?

Obviously the answer to both of these questions is no. Experts currently believe that diabetics can eat anything they wish, as long as they plan properly and follow certain rules. They also believe that if everybody ate according to the guidelines put forth for diabetics, many Americans would be a lot healthier. For there's really no such thing as a "diabetic diet"—there are only some basic rules for sensible eating that hold true for everyone, whether they have diabetes or not.

One thing is true: because these rules require a fairly dramatic change in the average American way of eating, they're difficult to follow all the time. Most nondiabetics can get away with slipups, although an imprudent diet will take its toll over the years. For a diabetic, however, the stakes are higher. Diabetics must plan their meals carefully to prevent their blood sugar from varying too dramatically. Many doctors claim that careful control of the diet is the single most important factor in the successful management of diabetes. And there's a bonus: many diabetics find that their disease can be managed *through diet alone.* Nemesis and guardian angel—to many diabetics, diet is both.

THE BENEFITS OF A SENSIBLE DIET

Through diet you can diminish the peaks and valleys in your blood glucose level. This has several benefits:

- It delays or even completely prevents complications.

- It maintains energy and a feeling of well-being and diminishes feelings of weakness or fatigue.

- Through its beneficial effect on metabolism a normal blood glucose level helps maintain normal levels of other nutrients, especially amino acids (the components of protein), ketone bodies (the byproducts of fat metabolism, discussed in Chapter One), and fat.

Other advantages of a healthy diet include:

- a decreased risk of heart disease, which in diabetics is particularly high

- the maintenance of ideal body weight, which is all many Type II diabetics need to control their diabetes

Tips for Successful Diet Therapy

1. Find a good dietitian or nutritionist. He or she is just as important a part of your management team as your physician. Good communication with your dietitian is essential so she can design a diet that accommodates your personal taste as well as your life-style and medical needs.

   When you plan your first visit, the nutritionist will probably tell you to record everything you eat and drink for the one to three days before your appointment. This will give her an idea of your eating patterns, your favorite foods, and the circumstances under which you eat (frequent business lunches, for example). Many doctors or clinics specializing in diabetes treatment have dietitians on staff. If yours doesn't, contact a local hospital or the American Dietetic Association in Chicago. (The phone number is given in Chapter Eight.) Make sure the person you consult is a registered dietitian (often referred to as simply RD), which means he or she is certified by the American Dietetic Association.

2. Stay abreast of new developments in all aspects of diabetes care. Read books, take courses, join support groups—do everything you can to remain knowledgeable.

3. Set goals with your dietitian. For example, for someone who's not hungry in the morning, eating breakfast may be a goal.

4. Visit the dietitian periodically—no less than once a year —for a reassessment of your diet and your needs. See her more often if your life changes in some way. For

example, you may get a new job that alters your schedule and thus changes your eating habits. You should also plan ahead for any trips you may be taking or for any other situation that affects your normal eating pattern.

5. Develop a plan for sick days and emergencies. Don't let yourself be caught unaware!

CURRENT KNOWLEDGE ABOUT DIET FOR THE DIABETIC

The use of diet to treat diabetes goes back thousands of years. Those of us living in the age of insulin may find it difficult to imagine the plight of earlier scientists, but remember that they had to manage diabetic patients without knowing what caused the disease. What they *did* know was that these patients accumulated sugar in their urine and their blood. From this observation came two schools of thought. One stated that, because diabetics lost sugar in their body fluids, they should be given more carbohydrate to replenish it. The second school declared it was better to maintain diabetics on less, rather than more, carbohydrate, because they had an excess already—otherwise why would it spill out in the urine and blood? The second group seems to have prevailed over the centuries, and thus developed the belief that carbohydrate is poison to the diabetic. This idea persists in many quarters today, despite decades of evidence that diabetics respond well to a balanced diet with a generous allotment of complex carbohydrate.

Some Facts about Digestion

When doctors talk about "carbohydrate," they're referring
to a large group of foods that includes starches and sugars.
Chemically these items are similar; the major difference is
that starch is made up of long chains of sugar molecules
that are linked together in food and separated during digestion. For this reason starches are often described as "complex carbohydrates," and their sugar components are called
"simple sugars."

When you eat something that contains starch—a piece of
bread, for example—it's broken down in the body to simple
sugars, which are then absorbed into the bloodstream,
causing blood glucose to rise. In the nondiabetic individual
the pancreas detects this rise in blood sugar and responds
by releasing more insulin, which helps the glucose leave
the blood and enter the cells of various organs, to be used
as fuel or stored. This is a highly simplified explanation of
the role of insulin in regulating blood sugar.

Because it takes time for the body to break them down,
the complex carbohydrates allow a relatively steady trickle
of sugar into the blood after you've eaten a meal. Thus they
don't raise blood sugar too quickly or too much. Simple
sugar, on the other hand, like the sugar you find in jams,
jellies, or soft drinks, enters the blood rapidly because it
doesn't have to go through the digestive process—it's already been broken down. So a heavy dose of sugar, like
that found in a can of soda, enters the blood almost immediately and causes a dramatic rise in blood sugar. This is no
problem for people who don't have diabetes, because they
can respond with a suitable outpouring of insulin that brings

blood sugar back to an acceptable level. But for diabetics such a rapid rise in blood sugar can spell disaster.

Today most experts agree that a good "diabetic diet" is one that contains plenty of complex carbohydrate. According to the American Diabetes Association fifty-five to sixty percent of your daily calories should be derived from carbohydrate—the same recommendations made for everyone else. This will help regulate your blood sugar, maintain your energy, and generally help keep you feeling good.

The Glycemic Index

If you've already done some reading on the subject of diabetes, you may have encountered something known as the "glycemic index." This refers to the effect of different foods, usually complex carbohydrates, on blood-glucose levels over a period of time. Researchers have discovered that, among foods containing the same amount of carbohydrate, some raise blood-glucose levels more than others. Bread and potatoes have the highest glycemic index—that is, they seem to raise blood glucose the most—while lentils and pasta have the lowest glycemic index. Some doctors now advise their diabetic patients to emphasize foods with a low glycemic index.

In fact, however, the glycemic index is a controversial entity. According to a 1986 conference conducted by the National Institutes of Health (NIH), a food's glycemic index may vary depending on methods of cooking, storing, and processing the food, as well as genetic differences in digestion and even how thoroughly you chew! In addition a food's glycemic index may change when the food is consumed as part of a meal with other ingredients. For these reasons the NIH experts did not recommend the use of the glycemic index when formulating a diabetic diet.

The Sweet Truth about Sugar

As a diabetic you've undoubtedly been told, time and again, to abolish sugar from your diet. And there's no question that, when consumed by itself as the only sweetener, particularly on an empty stomach, sugar will be rapidly absorbed and raise blood glucose too much.

At the same time, however, doctors and dietitians have finally come to realize that their diabetic patients are only human. It's the rare person who can give up her favorite foods entirely, and it's the even rarer individual who isn't—at least occasionally—tempted by something sweet. So now, after observing that patients can consume modest quantities of sugar without dire results, the American Diabetes Association and the American Dietetic Association allow sugar to compose up to five percent of the carbohydrate calories in a diabetic diet. That means, if you consume about one thousand calories' worth of carbohydrate per day —which isn't so much if you're eating eighteen hundred to two thousand calories altogether—up to fifty of those calories can come from sugar. That's the equivalent of about three teaspoons of sugar, or about four ounces of cola. Not much, perhaps, but enough to add a little more variety to your diet.

The Role of Fiber

Along with starch and simple sugars your diet contains another form of carbohydrate: fiber. The human body cannot digest fiber, so it passes through unabsorbed. Nevertheless this carbohydrate plays an important role in the diet by keeping us regular and possibly by lowering our risks of colon cancer and heart disease. There's also evidence that fiber may prevent blood sugar from climbing too high after a meal, although not all doctors are convinced that this is true.

Food contains two kinds of fiber: soluble and insoluble. Soluble fiber, the kind thought to affect blood sugar, is found in fruits, vegetables, and oat bran. Nuts, seeds, and legumes are also good sources of soluble fiber. As its name implies, soluble fiber absorbs water and becomes a gellike substance during digestion. In addition to moderating blood sugar this form of fiber is thought to help lower the risk of heart disease. Here again, however, there's been some controversy.

Insoluble fiber occurs in whole grains and wheat bran. This is the kind of fiber thought to lower colon-cancer risk, but it doesn't appear to influence blood sugar or the risk of heart disease. So for maximum health benefits your diet should contain both soluble and insoluble fiber.

DIETARY RECOMMENDATIONS

So far this discussion has emphasized carbohydrate, but that isn't all you consume in an average meal. Your body needs protein to manufacture hormones and enzymes and rebuild worn-out tissue, while fat serves as another important energy source and as a carrier for several vitamins. Fat also helps regulate the process of digestion, further ensuring that the food you eat trickles into the blood at a moderate rate so that your blood sugar doesn't skyrocket.

Clearly, then, the best diet for you is one that contains protein, fat, and complex carbohydrates in the right proportions. That's why the American Dietetic Association, the American Diabetic Association, the National Resource Council, the American Heart Association, and several other national health organizations have endorsed the following recommendations, which are the same for diabetics as they are for anyone else.

1. Fifty-five to sixty percent of all daily calories should come from carbohydrate, with sugar (sucrose) contributing not more than five percent of those calories. The rest of your carbohydrate should come from starchy foods like potatoes and whole-grain pasta, cereal, and breads.

2. Less than thirty percent of all daily calories should come from fat, of which not more than ten percent should be from saturated fat. Good sources of unsaturated fat include corn, safflower, cottonseed, soybean, or sunflower oil.

3. Protein should contribute twelve to twenty percent of a day's calories. Good sources of lean protein include white meat poultry without the skin, nonfat milk and dairy products, and fish.

4. We should consume thirty-five to forty grams of fiber per day. A slice of whole-wheat bread contains about two grams; a bowl of oatmeal, about four. A cup of bran

cereal has over twenty grams; an apple and half a grape-fruit each have roughly three.

5. Cholesterol consumption should average less than three hundred milligrams per day, slightly more than that found in the yolk of a large egg.

6. Salt consumption should be less than three thousand milligrams per day. One teaspoon of salt contains more than two thousand milligrams. Some TV dinners provide you with a day's worth of salt in one sitting.

DIET TIPS FOR DIABETICS

If you're accustomed to eating like most Americans, you may find these recommendations hard to put into practice. Some of them may even surprise you: eat *more* carbohydrate? *less* protein? Such advice runs counter to the diet information Americans have been hearing for years. Yet the fact is that experts now believe that a diet high in starchy foods like whole-grain pasta and bread, abundant in fresh fruits and vegetables, and relatively limited in protein and fat, is the healthiest one to have. Here are some suggestions to help you follow the diet recommendations. Remember, most of these tips hold true for anyone who wants to improve his or her nutrition.

1. Eat less fat. Fatty foods include butter, cream, whole milk, mayonnaise, and many cheeses.

2. Eat more complex carbohydrates, especially those high in fiber.

3. Eat less sugar.

4. Use less salt.

5. Make sure your portions are correct. Weigh and measure your food until you know what an adequate portion looks like.

6. Read labels; be on the alert for ingredients like salt or sweeteners such as fructose, sorbitol, or mannitol. These sugars can raise your blood sugar too high if you're not careful. They also add unnecessary calories to many foods.

EXCHANGE LISTS

The best way to ensure you're getting a healthy diet is to work with your dietitian to develop a meal plan that's right for you. This plan will allow you to choose from six food groups for each meal and snack. Because the foods in each group can be exchanged for one another, the groups have come to be known as exchange lists.

The foods in each exchange list are roughly equivalent in the quantities of carbohydrate, protein, fat, and calories they contain. The fact that they're interchangeable allows you to enjoy considerable variety and flexibility in your meals while still following your meal plan. This, in turn, increases the likelihood that you'll adhere to the plan the dietitian has designed.

The six exchange lists are:

• meat and meat substitutes (protein)

• starches and bread

• vegetables

- fruits

- milk

- fat

One exchange from each group provides the following nutrients:

Meat: seven grams protein, three grams fat, fifty-five calories* (example: one ounce of chicken without the skin, one ounce of lamb, or one-quarter cup canned tuna = one meat exchange)

Starch: fifteen grams carbohydrate, two grams protein, seventy calories (example: one slice of whole-wheat bread or three-quarters cup unsweetened cold cereal = one starch exchange)

Vegetables: five grams carbohydrate, two grams protein, twenty-five calories (example: one-half cup of asparagus, broccoli, or cauliflower = one vegetable exchange)

Fruit: ten grams carbohydrate, forty calories (example: one small apple or one-half cup orange juice = one fruit exchange)

Milk: twelve grams carbohydrate, eight grams protein, eighty calories** (example: one cup skim milk or unflavored skim milk [nonfat] yogurt = one milk exchange)

* These figures are for low-fat meat exchanges. Other cuts of meat might be considered medium or high fat. They have more calories and would contribute one-half or one fat exchange to the diet, respectively.
** Low-fat and whole milk have more calories and would contribute one-half to two fat exchanges, depending on the product used.

Fat: five grams fat, forty-five calories (example: one teaspoon of corn oil or ten almonds = one fat exchange)

Depending on your needs and tastes, your nutritionist can work with the exchange groups to develop a daily meal plan for you. For example, if you eat fruit but hate vegetables, for you a typical day's program for twelve hundred calories might include: six protein exchanges; six starch/bread exchanges; four fat exchanges; three fruit exchanges; two milk exchanges; and one vegetable exchange. The following chart illustrates a sample day's meals, based on this plan.

By using the lists and following your meal plan, you'll be able to control your daily intake of carbohydrate, protein, and fat, and balance your food and insulin. It's through this balance that you'll achieve good blood sugar control.

TIPS FOR TYPE I AND TYPE II DIABETICS

While the basic nutritional recommendations for each type of patient are the same, the goals for dietary therapy differ. Type I diabetics must coordinate their meals with their insulin injections so that their blood glucose always remains within safe boundaries. Type II diabetics often don't require any medication at all when they follow a proper diet. Frequently obese, these patients usually find that they can control their disease simply by losing weight and maintaining it within safe limits. Thus, a diet for the Type II diabetic usually concentrates first on getting her to achieve her ideal weight, and then on helping her stay there.

A SAMPLE MENU FOR ONE DAY

Meal	Starch/Bread	Meat	Fat	Fruit	Milk	Vegetables
			Servings per Exchange			
Breakfast						
3/4 cup cornflakes	1					
1 cup skim milk					1	
1/2 cup orange juice				1		
coffee						
Snack						
1 slice whole wheat toast	1					
1 teaspoon butter			1			
Lunch						
3 oz. chicken breast		3				
1 roll	2					
1 tablespoon mayonnaise			2			
2 leaves lettuce						Free
Tomato slices (1/2 tomato)						0.5
1 apple				1		
Snack						
1 1/2 cup popcorn, no butter	0.5					
1/2 cup skim milk					0.5	
Dinner						
3 oz. hamburger		3				
1/2 cup broccoli						0.5
1 teaspoon butter			1			
1/2 cup corn	1					
1/2 9-in. banana				1		
Bedtime Snack						
1 1/2 cup popcorn, no butter	0.5					
1/2 cup skim milk					0.5	
Total Servings/Exchange	6	6	4	3	2	1
Total Calories/Exchange	420	330	180	120	180	25
Total Daily Calories	1255					

Tips for Type I

1. Consistency is the cornerstone of your dietary therapy. You should eat your meals and snacks at the same time each day, and they should consist of the same number of exchanges from each list, according to your meal plan. This is the most important factor in achieving optimal blood-glucose control.

2. Remember to consider exercise when balancing your insulin and meals. (For more information on exercise please see the end of this chapter.)

3. Gradually increase the amount of fiber you consume. While many experts have questioned the evidence that it helps control your blood sugar and may lower your heart disease risk, there's no question that high-fiber foods are also usually high in the complex carbohydrates you need for energy. Do your SMBG more frequently as you add more fiber to see if you need any changes in your insulin dose.

4. If you're underweight, you may find that controlling your diabetes through diet, exercise, and insulin automatically helps you gain. If not, increasing the portions on your meal plan may help you gain while still eating balanced meals. Make sure your registered dietitian approves of this step.

5. Occasionally the Type I diabetic may become overweight. This may occur through overzealous use of insulin, or excessive food intake to counteract or avoid an insulin reaction. All of this indicates that a reevaluation of insulin dosing is in order. A Type I diabetic may also

develop poor eating habits when his blood glucose is
poorly controlled and he grows accustomed to feeling
hungry no matter how much he eats. When his blood
sugar is finally controlled, such a patient has already
developed the habit of eating too much, and so gains
weight.

The best plan here is probably to eat smaller portions
on one's usual meal plan. However, Type I patients who
wish to reduce should consult a dietitian before they do
so. Under no circumstances should they attempt a fad
diet like one of the liquid-protein regimes.

6. You may drink alcohol on occasion. If you enjoy wine
with your meal or a drink before dinner, ask your dietitian for the best way to incorporate it into your meal
plan. Most experts believe that half a glass of wine
(about two ounces) or the alcohol equivalent in gin,
Scotch, or other distilled spirits, once or twice a week,
is permissible for most diabetics. Avoid alcohol, however, until your blood-glucose levels are well under control, or if the level of certain fats in your blood, called
triglycerides, is too high. Pregnant women should also
not imbibe.

7. If you're the parent of a child or adolescent with Type I
diabetes, make sure your child visits the dietitian at
least once a year, and preferably every six months. Poor
blood-glucose control or improper diet may, in severe
cases, stunt a child's growth.

Tips for Type II

1. Lose weight! This is the single most important tip for the Type II diabetic who is obese. Your dietitian will develop the best weight-reduction plan for you, but in general the best way to cut calories is to cut out high-fat foods like butter, mayonnaise, many cheeses, ice cream, and some cuts of red meat. Instead fill up on "free" foods like salad greens, celery, cucumbers, cabbage, mushrooms, and zucchini. A sensible exercise program will also help you burn calories, and may help regulate your blood sugar as well. Fad diets, on the other hand, are as ill advised for you as they are for the Type I diabetic.

2. Adding more fiber to your diet may help you fill up faster.

3. Space your calories as evenly as possible throughout the day to avoid a heavy influx of calories at one time. Such a caloric concentration might overwhelm your body's limited capacity to metabolize food.

ALCOHOL AND SNACKS: A FEW WORDS ABOUT EACH

Alcohol

Perhaps you were surprised to read earlier that alcohol is permitted in the diabetic diet. The fact is, alcohol in small quantities isn't harmful, as long as your blood glucose is under good control. In fact, if a drink once or twice a week allows you to feel less deprived, it may help in the long run by encouraging you to follow your meal plan. Just remember a couple of precautions:

1. Do not drink on an empty stomach. If you have your cocktail at mealtime, eat something with it; if you drink late at night, have a bedtime snack. Remember that a drink or two may diminish your capacity to recognize and compensate for a hypoglycemic reaction if you take insulin or oral hypoglycemics; this possibility may be nipped in the bud if you routinely eat something, preferably containing protein or complex carbohydrates, when you imbibe.

2. Avoid sweet mixed drinks, cordials, and liqueurs, because of their high sugar content.

Snacks

Wisely planned snacks may help you avoid wide swings in blood sugar between meals. Your nutritionist can advise you on which snacks fit best into your meal plan and calorie level. A few tips:

1. Carbohydrate, even of the complex variety, may not last long enough in snack portions to have a significant effect on your blood sugar. Make sure your snacks include some protein and fat.

2. Type II diabetics taking oral hypoglycemics should snack between meals and at bedtime.

3. If you take regular insulin, have a snack two and a half hours after your injection. Patients taking intermediate insulin should plan a snack seven hours later.

SOME TIPS FOR SICK DAYS

Sick days can be a problem for the diabetic because blood sugar may fluctuate unpredictably when you're not feeling well. Ideally you should work out a plan in advance with your doctor and dietitian, not only for meals and snacks but for any necessary changes in medication. Here are some basic tips to keep in mind:

1. Take your usual insulin dose unless you have any other instructions from your doctor.

2. Test your blood glucose regularly. It's also a good idea to test your urine for ketones.

3. Drink plenty of liquids.

4. Sips of soft drinks, fruit juice, or sweetened tea may help the patient who can't keep food down, as might Popsicles, gelatin (with sugar), or sherbet.

5. If you can't keep *anything* down, notify your doctor immediately.

SOME THOUGHTS ON EXERCISE

Exercise offers some clear benefits to the diabetic, including:

- Weight loss if you are overweight, weight gain if you are underweight

- Decreased risk of heart disease, achieved through weight loss, lower levels of dangerous blood fats, strengthening of the heart, and lower blood pressure

- Relief from feelings of tension and stress

You may have also heard that regular exercise helps control blood-sugar levels by improving glucose tolerance and, possibly, by increasing the number of insulin receptors on muscle cells. There's no question that exercise increases glucose uptake by the muscles and so lowers blood glucose in the short term, but its beneficial long-term effects on blood sugar have been disputed. Many experts today describe them as "small but significant." But on the whole, exercise imparts real benefits to the diabetic—both Type I and Type II—and should be a regular part of everyone's routine.

Exercise Precautions for the Diabetic

People with diabetes can participate in any activity they wish, as long as they take a few precautions.

1. *It is absolutely essential to check with your doctor before starting any exercise program.* Tell him or her what you want to do, how often, and how much time you'll spend doing it.

2. It's also a good idea to ask your dietitian for any suggestions he or she might have regarding changes in diet on days that you exercise.

3. Start any new exercise routine slowly, and gradually build up to the level you want to attain. If you go running, for example, start with a routine of slow running for three to five minutes, then walking for a few minutes, then running slowly again. Build up gradually to a nonstop jog for twenty to thirty minutes.

4. Stop whenever you don't feel well. If necessary have some sugar, like a piece of candy or a soft drink. If you can, measure your blood glucose.

5. Try to make your exercise routine consistent—approximately the same amount each day.

6. If you're planning an active day—a long bike ride, for example—eat a larger-than-usual meal before, with extra protein and carbohydrate. Take a supply of sugar with you, such as candy or one of the emergency forms of glucose. Some diabetics find they have to take some extra sugar as often as every twenty to thirty minutes during prolonged exercise. If you can, it's also a good idea to check your blood glucose while you're exercising. Even better, call your doctor and dietitian before the event and ask for their suggestions.

DIET AND DIABETES: CONCLUSION

As you've seen, the "diabetic diet" is the same as a healthy diet for anyone else. Unfortunately nondiabetics can get away with more "cheating" than you can—although the consequences of a poor diet eventually catch up with many people, in the form of heart disease, obesity, and possibly even cancer. But for you the results are more immediate:

the loss of good blood-sugar control. Diabetics must try to anticipate each day's activities and plan their meals and snacks accordingly. They also have to be sure their food is in the proper balance and portions. Without question there are drawbacks to this way of life, primarily in the loss of spontaneity that's required to make your diet work. But isn't that a small price to pay if you can maintain good blood glucose control, avoid complications, and feel great?

FIVE

A DAY IN THE LIFE OF TWO DIABETICS

If much of the information in this book is new to you, you may be finding it difficult to see how some of this advice is put into practice, or how real diabetics manage in emergencies. Let's take two hypothetical people with diabetes and see how they cope with blood sugar that's too high or too low. Each of these people is a composite of several real diabetic patients. As you read these accounts, remember that diabetes management must be tailored to each individual: what works for someone else may not work for you.

ROBERTA M.

Roberta is an obese fifty-year-old public relations executive with a stressful job and a demanding schedule. She's had Type II diabetes for five years. Usually, Roberta can control her blood sugar through diet alone, but her doctor knows her job is difficult; he also knows that Roberta sometimes forgets about the careful planning her disease requires. He has advised her to keep some emergency insulin on hand at home and in the office, and has prescribed an algorithm to follow if she needs it.

Right now Roberta is undergoing even more stress than usual, because her company is fighting to keep a very important account. Here's how she got through a recent day.

6:00 A.M.: SMBG. Blood glucose is high at 160 mg/dl. Roberta promises herself to take up aerobics when the crunch is over at work. Breakfast: A bagel with diet margarine, about six ounces of orange juice, and coffee with half-and-half.

7:30 A.M.: Arrive at office; work straight through until 12:30, including a tense meeting with her boss about the status of her account.

12:30 P.M.: Meeting over, Roberta feels thirsty and nauseated. Nibbles on a tuna fish sandwich; has a few pieces of candy brought in by a coworker and several glasses of water; nothing else.

1:00 P.M.–2:30 P.M.: Back to work. Must stop several times to go to the water cooler. Has some more orange juice; still feels queasy.

3:00 P.M.: Feeling worse, Roberta tests her blood glucose. At 320 mg/dl, it's frighteningly high. She takes some of her emergency insulin as instructed in her algorithm and starts feeling better within a half hour.

4:30 P.M.: Blood glucose is down to 280. Roberta takes more insulin.

6:30 P.M.: Roberta's blood glucose is now down to 200, which is approaching a safe range. She takes one more shot of insulin.

7:30 P.M.: Blood glucose is 175. Roberta feels better and resumes working. Chastened by her frightening experience, she orders in a balanced dinner of broiled chicken, string beans, and a baked potato. She eats over her work and stays in the office until 10:00 P.M., a typical day for her.

Roberta's experience illustrates the fact that stress raises blood sugar. Along with having her keep insulin on hand for emergencies such as this, Roberta's doctor has told her that exercise and proper nutrition can help her lose weight, control her diabetes, and alleviate some of her stress. After years of nagging, she's finally made a few changes in her life-style, but she tends to put aside her own well-being when the demands of her job become extreme.

LARRY B.

Larry is a nineteen-year-old college student who's had diabetes since the age of four. After all these years he's become pretty good at controlling his blood sugar and handling emergencies, but he's not invulnerable to unforeseen events. Here's a page out of his diary:

7:30 A.M.: SMBG. Blood glucose is 110 mg/dl, a safe level. Larry takes his insulin and has breakfast: orange juice, cold cereal with skim milk, one slice of whole wheat toast with diet margarine, coffee with skim milk.

8:00 A.M.: Running late, Larry jogs to his first class.

8:15 A.M.–10:30 A.M.: Classes.

10:30 A.M.: Larry takes a break. Buys a banana and an iced tea at the campus coffee shop, but gets into a heated discussion with a friend over something said in class, and neglects to eat the banana.

11:00 A.M.–1:00 P.M.: Classes.

1:15 P.M.: Suddenly very hungry, Larry hurries to the cafeteria for lunch. He has a roast beef sandwich on rye bread with lettuce and tomato, potato chips, a glass of skim milk, and half of the banana left over from his snack.

2:00 P.M.–4:00 P.M.: Classes.

4:30 P.M.–5:30 P.M.: Larry's roommate and some friends persuade him to join in an impromptu game of touch football. Larry knows he should go home and test his blood sugar first, but he's eager for a break from his day of classes, and decides to play spontaneously just this once.

5:45 P.M.: Larry runs to the library to get the last copy of a book he needs for a paper he's writing. Walking down the library steps he feels a sudden wave of fatigue. Headachy and weak in the knees, he momentarily collapses on the steps. Somehow he's able to go back into the library, where there's a soda machine. He buys a can of cola (the kind made with sugar) and feels better within a few minutes after drinking it.

6:00 P.M.: SMBG reveals that Larry's blood sugar is 80 mg/dl.

7:00 P.M.: Larry's predinner blood glucose reading is 140, back within a safe range.

10:00 P.M.: Blood glucose is now 160. Larry takes his usual evening insulin shot and prepares for bed.

A diabetic since early childhood, Larry has learned how to handle his disease and lead a normal life. In general, his blood glucose is under good control. Nevertheless, there are times when he slips up, and this was one of them. The brisk walk to his first class, the forgotten midmorning snack, the football game, and the afternoon run to the library all lowered Larry's blood sugar too much, putting him in the early stages of hypoglycemia. Fortunately, Larry was experienced enough to recognize the symptoms and do something about them immediately. This close call did teach him, however, never to take chances: from now on he'll do his SMBG and make appropriate adjustments in his food or insulin dose before participating in an activity like football, even if it means entering the game a little late. In this case, for example, he could have eaten a light snack before playing. Even the banana half left over from the morning would have been better than nothing.

SIX

THE COMPLICATIONS OF DIABETES

As a diabetic, you may have heard about patients who have gone blind, suffered amputations, been placed on kidney dialysis, or endured some other horrible fate. This does indeed happen to an unfortunate few, but the good news is that today most diabetics can avoid the worst consequences of their disease. Strong evidence suggests that consistent maintenance of blood glucose within normal limits—something doctors like to refer to as tight control—may delay the appearance of many complications and minimize them when they do occur. It may even be able to prevent them entirely. So the information here is presented, not to frighten you, but to impress upon you the importance of good diabetic control, combined with a few precautions and regular checkups—particularly of the most vulnerable areas: the eyes, heart and blood vessels, and feet.

The statistics of diabetic complications are indeed grim. Because it involves defects in the most fundamental aspects of metabolism, diabetes affects virtually every organ system in the body. What's more, its effects are cumulative, so the longer you have diabetes, the greater your chances of experiencing one or more complications. Diabetes is the number-one cause of blindness among adults in the United States and ranks sixth as a direct cause of death. If you considered the deaths caused by the complications, diabetes would be the third greatest cause of death in this country. In addition diabetes is held responsible for over fifty percent of the amputations performed annually and twenty-five percent of all kidney failure.

In most cases diabetic complications have few or no symptoms until they've progressed to a severe stage. Sometimes the early symptoms they do present are diagnosed as something else. But they all have one feature in common: poor control of the patient's diabetes, and the persistent high blood-sugar levels that go along with it. In general people with Type I diabetes run a higher risk of developing complications than Type II patients, possibly because the Type I patient usually has the disease longer. Complications are most common in people who have had diabetes for fifteen to twenty years or more. But it's important to remember that there's no guarantee you'll get them: many diabetics never develop any complications at all. In other patients it's not uncommon to see problems occur in several organs. But few people develop them everywhere.

DIABETIC NEUROPATHY

The most common diabetic complication is neuropathy, or damage to the nerves. Doctors still don't entirely understand how or why this condition occurs, but its symptoms may range from mild but annoying to incapacitating pain.

On a more positive note neuropathy often abates after a few months or years.

Nerves damaged by neuropathy no longer transmit impulses normally, so that symptoms may vary at different times in the same patient. At one moment the affected area may hurt unbearably, while at other times it may itch, tingle, burn, or just go numb. These sensations come and go unpredictably but seem to occur most often at night. Because neuropathy takes such an unpredictable course, many doctors first diagnose its symptoms as something else.

Neuropathy may take two basic forms. Peripheral neuropathy results from damage to the nerves governing parts of the body under more or less conscious control, like the arms and legs. Autonomic neuropathy affects nerves serving involuntary functions, like digestion or perspiration.

Peripheral Neuropathy

The early symptoms of peripheral neuropathy include loss of feeling in the affected area, pain or tingling in the hands or feet, and loss of normal reflexes. It strikes the legs and feet most often; many patients report feeling as if they're walking on pillows or clouds, or on wood. Peripheral neuropathy may also increase sensitivity to touch, to the extent that some patients experience pain when covered by a bedsheet.

Peripheral neuropathy seems to get worse in cold or wet weather. Fortunately its torments frequently go away within a few months, although few patients would be comforted by knowing that the worse the pain, the more quickly the condition may subside.

One of the worst consequences of peripheral neuropathy is the development of neuropathic ulcers, sores that occur on pressure points of the feet. Usually the ulcer begins as a small blister or bruise that goes unnoticed due to loss of sensation in the feet. Eventually a callus may form, under which an ulcer may develop. Neuropathic ulcers must be treated immediately, to keep them from growing or becoming infected. In addition pressure on the feet must be minimized by having patients wear special devices in their shoes and by staying off their feet as much as possible.

Do not underestimate the seriousness of a bruise on your foot. In diabetics untreated foot sores and ulcers are ripe for infection, which may develop into gangrene if not caught early. Examine your feet daily and have your doctor check them at every visit.

Autonomic Neuropathy

Less common than peripheral neuropathy, autonomic neuropathy may lead to symptoms such as:

- orthostatic hypotension, an abrupt drop in blood pressure that occurs upon standing suddenly, which leads to feelings of dizziness or lightheadedness

- abnormal sweating patterns on the face or feet

- changes in the muscle or bone structure of the feet

- abdominal pain

- sexual impotence in men or other sexual problems

- the inability to feel a full bladder, leading to urine backup into the kidneys or incomplete bladder emptying, either of which may promote infections and, ultimately, serious kidney damage

- digestive problems, such as diarrhea

When to Suspect Neuropathy

Early neuropathy may have no symptoms at all, or the symptoms may be so variable that the doctor may first think they indicate some other disorder. You can, however, take a few precautions:

1. At the first sign of any changes in sensation in your feet, tell your doctor *instantly*. Also check your feet regularly and get prompt treatment for any bruises, blisters, calluses, or sores, no matter how insignificant they may seem.

2. Tell your doctor if you start urinating less frequently, or if urine volume falls off. The physician can prescribe drugs to restore your normal pattern or may tell you to urinate every few hours whether or not you feel the urge, in an effort to prevent both urine buildup and urinary-tract infections.

3. If you suspect you may have developed a urinary-tract infection, get treatment immediately and maintain it for as long as your doctor instructs.

4. It cannot be emphasized enough: *Maintain good blood-glucose control.*

Treatment of Neuropathy

Currently most physicians treat painful neuropathies with painkillers and tranquilizers to help patients sleep. Some doctors also prescribe antidepressants and mood elevators.

Recently diabetes researchers have been encouraged by experiments with a class of drugs known as aldose reductase inhibitors. These products seem to relieve neuropathy by altering one of the metabolic defects thought responsible for the development of nerve damage. While more research is needed, the aldose reductase inhibitors appear to hold promise in the treatment of diabetic neuropathy. And remember: Good blood-glucose control may help you avoid many, if not all, of the manifestations of neuropathy.

MICROVASCULAR CHANGES

Experts currently believe that many complications arise at least in part because of damage to the blood vessels that serve the various organs. Studies conducted on humans and experimental animals have shown a thickening in portions of tiny blood vessels that is proportional to the duration of the disease. These microvascular changes, as they are called, have been found even before any other complications appear. While these findings have been most obvious in the kidney, they've also occurred in other tissue such as muscle. That these changes are somehow related to the metabolic defects in diabetes has been borne out by observations that diabetic patients who receive kidney transplants from nondiabetic donors develop the same complications within a few years.

MACROVASCULAR CHANGES

Changes also occur in the larger blood vessels, like the big arteries that serve the heart. These changes resemble the normal "hardening of the arteries" that occurs with aging, the difference being that in diabetics they're far more extensive and happen much earlier in life. In fact some experts have suggested that diabetic complications may be somehow related to an accelerated aging process. There's no proof to this theory yet, but there is some evidence to support it, and it's an intriguing area for future research.

Your risk of developing microvascular or macrovascular complications is increased by these factors:

- cigarette smoking

- high blood pressure (hypertension)

- high levels of certain fats in the blood

- lack of exercise

- poor blood-glucose control

COMPLICATIONS OF THE SKIN

It's long been known that diabetics are more prone to complications of the skin, such as:

- boils

- sties

- inflammation around the nails

- dry, itchy skin, often causing persistent scratching, which results in irritation and possible infection of the area

- athlete's foot

- fungal infections of the mouth, such as thrush

- yeast infections in the vagina, the groin (in men), the anus (in either sex), or around the armpits or between fingers or toes

- slow healing of bruises or cuts

- spotting or discoloration, especially on the skin of the shins and lower legs, usually resulting from breakage of small blood vessels in these areas

Skin problems often result from poor diabetic control and are sometimes the first sign that you have diabetes at all. When you have an open sore, no matter how shallow or small, the blood's high sugar content invites the proliferation of infecting organisms. The metabolic defects of diabetes also affect your immune response and ability to heal.

Fortunately, when treated promptly, most cases of diabetic skin lesions heal completely and do not produce more serious complications.

Treatment of Skin Complications

1. Tell your doctor about any cut that's infected or slow to heal, as well as about any boils, athlete's foot, or any abnormal vaginal discharge.

2. Keep your skin scrupulously clean. Ask your doctor or nurse to teach you the proper care for minor cuts and bruises.

Skin-Care Dos and Don'ts

1. Do protect your skin against drying or chapping, since this may dehydrate it or invite bacterial invasion.

2. Do wear scarves and warm gloves when it's cold.

3. Do use products like moisturizers, lotions, and superfatted soaps to prevent drying of the skin; if you live in a cold, dry climate, do use a humidifier in your home.

4. Do wet your skin before applying moisturizers or oils to seal the moisture in.

5. Don't take too many baths, especially in cold weather.

6. Don't wash too often with soap.

7. Don't use solvents or disinfectants, like alcohol, on your skin.

COMPLICATIONS OF THE EYE

Diabetic eye complications include exacerbation of cataracts, problems in focusing, and retinal damage.

Cataracts

A cataract is a lens that clouds over, resulting in vision loss. Diabetes probably does not raise your risk of developing a cataract, but it may allow the cataract to progress more quickly once it does occur. Once again, the maintenance of safe blood-glucose levels may help slow a cataract's course. New drugs are also under development that may prevent diabetes-related cataracts by diminishing the buildup of sugar by-products in the lens.

Currently the best treatment for a severe cataract is to remove it. The operation is simple and fast, and many ophthalmologists perform it right in the office. If appropriate the doctor will replace your natural lens with an artificial one that he inserts in the eye during surgery.

Focusing Problems

Blurring, temporary double vision, and frequent changes of prescription are common in people with poorly controlled diabetes. That's because the lens in your eye, which normally focuses light on the retina, the light-sensitive tissue in back of the eye, may swell or shrink with fluctuating blood-sugar levels, impairing its ability to focus light. High blood sugar diminishes long-distance vision, while low blood sugar affects near vision or may produce double vision. So even if you get new glasses, you may find they're useless in a few days if your blood sugar isn't under control. Some doctors advise newly diagnosed diabetics to wait a month before getting new glasses, so that their blood-sugar levels are stable.

Retinopathy

The most common—and potentially most serious—diabetic visual problem is retinopathy, damage to the small blood vessels in the light-sensitive tissue in back of the eye. Approximately forty percent of all people with diabetes have at least mild signs of diabetic retinopathy; three percent experience severe visual loss. About half of all Type I diabetics develop some form of retinopathy after eight to ten years with diabetes; in Type II patients the figure is one in four. More than ten years after diagnosis over eighty percent of all diabetics may expect to develop some form of retinopathy. The patients at highest risk of visual problems include black women and those who developed diabetes in childhood.

Retinopathy develops from the gradual decrease in blood and oxygen flow to the retina, due to weakening of the tiny blood vessels found in the eye. These fragile vessels may bulge and break more easily, causing the leakage of blood and other fluid into the retina. To compensate for the loss of the blood vessels, new ones form, sometimes hemorrhaging themselves and sometimes reaching into other parts of the eye.

This entire process is painless and often elicits no symptoms, unless blood-vessel damage occurs near the macula, the portion of the retina responsible for sharp, clear vision, like that needed for reading or driving. The macula swells when fluid leaks into it, resulting in a condition known as macular edema. Macular edema, in turn, leads to blurred vision.

The vast majority of diabetics develop a mild condition known as background retinopathy, which requires regular checkups by an ophthalmologist and possibly special treatment, such as laser therapy. In all but a relatively few patients, background retinopathy gets no worse and sometimes even improves.

Proliferative Retinopathy

Some unfortunate patients go on to develop a condition known as proliferative retinopathy. The name arises from the extensive proliferation of blood vessels in the retina, which are as fragile as their predecessors. When these vessels break they bleed into the gellike substance that fills the eyeball (the vitreous humor) and normally helps transmit light from the lens to the retina. Small quantities of blood in the vitreous may dissipate with no problem, but in advanced proliferative retinopathy the bleeding may interfere with vision. In addition the rapid growth of new vessels and more bleeding promotes the formation of scar tissue, which may ultimately cause the retina to detach from the eye.

Proliferative retinopathy may progress for years with no symptoms, as long as it occurs on the periphery of the retina, away from the macula. But if it should reach the macula, or if too much blood enters the vitreous, or if the retina should detach, serious vision problems result. Blindness may occur from excess blood in the vitreous or extensive retinal damage.

Treatment of Retinopathy

The good news is that background and proliferative retinopathy are treatable, and the vast majority of patients, even those with an advanced form of the disease, do *not* go blind.

Currently the best treatment for retinopathy involves use of a laser, a special light beam the doctor aims at the leaking blood vessels in the eye. The laser seals off the leaks, preventing further visual decline. If parts of the retina have already been seriously damaged, the doctor may use the laser to remove them, sometimes reducing one's risk of severe visual loss by as much as sixty percent. In addition the laser may also be used to "glue" a detached retina back in place.

Some patients may undergo a vitrectomy, a procedure during which the doctor removes parts of the vitreous that have been stained with blood. The gel is replaced with saline solution. In many cases this operation may relieve the clouded vision that occurred when blood leaked into the vitreous.

Prevention of Visual Loss—
Dos and Don'ts

1. Do maintain your blood sugar within normal limits: 140 or less when fasting; 200 or less two hours after a meal. This is especially important during the first five years of your diabetes, since studies have shown careful control at this time to be particularly good at preventing retinal damage.

2. Do have yourself checked regularly for high blood pressure and get treatment for it if you must. High blood pressure greatly increases the risk of retinopathy.

3. Do have regular eye examinations, at least once a year but preferably every six months. Make sure your ophthalmologist knows you have diabetes. If your doctor has already diagnosed some background retinopathy, have your eyes checked every three months.

4. Do take special care to have your eyes checked regularly if you:

   • have had diabetes more than five years

   • are a diabetic woman who's pregnant or planning pregnancy

   • have a history of difficulty controlling your blood sugar

5. Do report any vision changes to your doctor *immediately.*

6. Don't wait until your vision changes to start getting your eyes checked.

7. Don't smoke.

8. Don't cancel or skip scheduled appointments for eye checkups. Doctors can now detect retinopathy in its earliest stages, greatly increasing their chances of heading off serious problems.

9. Don't start an exercise program without checking with your doctor first. If you haven't already developed retinopathy, exercise may help prevent it. But in people who already have retinopathy, an exercise-induced rise in blood pressure may trigger the breakage and bleeding of tiny blood vessels in the eye.

HEART AND BLOOD-VESSEL COMPLICATIONS

Heart disease is the number-one killer in America, and it's the number-one killer of diabetics. People with diabetes develop hardening of the arteries, especially in the heart, head, and legs, more often than other people and as much as a decade earlier. According to the U.S. Public Health Service cardiovascular disease—that is, heart and blood-vessel disease—accounts for fifty percent of the deaths in the general population, but seventy-five percent of the deaths in diabetics. Diabetics are twice as likely to have strokes and coronary heart disease—disease of the large arteries that serve the heart—and five times as likely to have blood-vessel disease of the extremities.

The steps for avoiding heart disease are the same for diabetics as they are for anyone else, with one addition: maintain good blood-sugar control. Beyond that the recommendations for preventing cardiovascular complications include:

1. Achieve and maintain normal body weight.

2. Keep your blood pressure under control. If your doctor prescribes blood-pressure medication, make sure he knows you have diabetes, because some blood-pressure drugs may be dangerous for diabetics.

3. Stop smoking.

4. Exercise regularly, but get your doctor's approval before starting an exercise program.

5. If your blood cholesterol is too high, try lowering it through diet, exercise, and medication. Doctors currently recommend that you try to keep your total blood cholesterol under 200 mg/dl. Once again, however, advise your doctor of your diabetes if he prescribes drugs, since some cholesterol-lowering medicines react poorly with oral hypoglycemics; others may increase the risk of retinal bleeding in some people.

KIDNEY COMPLICATIONS

When functioning properly blood vessels in the kidneys filter waste products from the blood while allowing glucose, protein, and other important items to remain in the circulation. The waste enters the urine and is excreted. Diabetic kidney disease occurs when those blood vessels become thickened or damaged, so they lose this filtering capacity and allow protein and glucose to escape into the urine.

Severe kidney damage is most often seen in people who

have had diabetes longer than ten to fifteen years. Apparently something about prolonged diabetes promotes thickening and damage of the kidney blood vessels. If allowed to progress, diabetic kidney damage may lead to uremia—the presence of excessive levels of waste products in the blood —and kidney failure.

Fortunately this kind of severe kidney damage occurs in less than half of all Type I diabetics, and in even fewer Type II patients. But, just as with the other complications, good glucose control and regular, thorough checkups may help lower your risk of kidney damage even more. These measures are especially important if you have high blood pressure or a tendency to develop urinary-tract infections (diabetics have a higher risk of both), which increase the likelihood of kidney complications.

Regular checkups are important because early kidney damage often has no symptoms. Even after protein starts to appear in the urine, which is one sign of kidney problems, a patient may experience no symptoms until eighty to ninety percent of his kidney function is lost, a process which may take several years.

What can you do to decrease your risk of kidney damage? Good blood-glucose control and treatment of high blood pressure are paramount. In fact there's some evidence that controlling your blood sugar may even diminish kidney damage after it's begun. Beyond that you should notify your doctor immediately if you experience problems emptying your bladder, if you see blood in your urine, or if you have any other reason to think you have kidney damage or a urinary-tract infection. If your doctor suspects kidney damage, he will perform several tests, including a measurement of the protein in your urine. You may be placed on a low-protein diet to make the kidneys' job a little easier and slow the progression of the damage.

If kidney damage is very severe, the physician may suggest dialysis or even a kidney transplant. Remember, though, that only a relatively few patients require these last-ditch measures, and that important strides have been made in these treatments in the past few years. Today survival rates among diabetics undergoing dialysis or kidney transplants is almost as good as that of nondiabetics who require these therapies. Nevertheless they are best avoided if at all possible. The best treatment for kidney damage is prevention.

COMPLICATIONS OF THE FEET

Some people have their heads in the clouds, but the thoughts of most diabetics focus down—on their feet. Foot problems are a constant source of worry to the diabetic, because, as you saw earlier in this chapter, the slightest blister or bump may become infected and usher in the possibility of all sorts of horrible developments, chiefly gangrene and the possibility of amputation. That's because peripheral neuropathy may cause a loss of sensation in the feet, so you can no longer feel if they're dangerously hot, cold, or wounded. Even major injuries may go unrecognized. Gangrene may set in when the feet are repeatedly traumatized, creating ulcers that are exacerbated by poor circulation that cannot deliver oxygen or immune cells, whose ability to fight off infection is already impaired. In addition, even if you take oral antibiotics that work by entering the blood and being delivered to the infection site, they won't be effectively delivered to the feet because of this compromised circulation. It's situations such as this that have made diabetes one of the leading causes of amputation in adults.

Don't become another statistic. Isn't it better to spend a few extra minutes, and even dollars, protecting your feet today to prevent serious complications tomorrow? Along with daily visual inspection of your feet, using a mirror on hard-to-see spots if necessary, you can take the following foot precautions, developed by the National Diabetes Advisory Board:

1. Keep your feet clean. Bathe them daily in warm (not hot) water. Dry carefully, especially between the toes.

2. Walking is the best exercise for your feet. There are also special exercises to stimulate circulation, if needed.

3. Give up smoking to preserve your good circulation.

4. Wear clean socks or stockings that fit properly.

5. Soft leather shoes or jogging (running) shoes, if your routine permits them, are best for daily wear. Shoes should be comfortable at the time of purchase. New shoes should be worn for short periods at first. Consult your physician or podiatrist about the best kind of shoes to buy, and what to look for in fit.

6. Cut toenails straight across and not too short. File calluses or corns carefully with emery boards only.

7. Avoid extremes of temperature, either hot or cold. Test water before bathing.

8. Do not walk barefoot or on hot surfaces such as sandy beaches and around swimming pools.

9. Do not use over-the-counter medicines for corns or blisters without checking with your doctor first.

10. Wear socks if your feet feel cold at night. Do not use hot-water bottles or heating pads.

11. Ask for help if you find it difficult to take care of your feet.

12. Make sure your feet are examined regularly by a physician or podiatrist.

13. Report injuries promptly and follow your practitioner's recommendations exactly.

14. Always check your shoes before putting them on. Look and feel inside to make sure there aren't any tacks, little pebbles, or anything else that might injure your feet.

15. Taking off your socks while waiting to see the doctor will remind him—and you—that your feet should be examined during the checkup.

CONCLUSION

It's true that diabetic complications may be devastating if they reach their worst stages, but most people can prevent this by taking the simple precaution of controlling their blood glucose. Remember: With the right planning and preparation, and frequent SMBG, you can minimize or avoid the disease's worst complications. In fact the planning and care required for blood-sugar control often means that diabetics take better care of themselves than the rest of the population. As a result some doctors claim that their diabetic patients may live longer than they might have if they'd never gotten the disease. So don't use the risk of complications as a reason to despair; instead, make it an incentive to lead the healthiest life you can.

SEVEN

DIABETES IN PEOPLE WITH SPECIAL NEEDS

Diabetes is an equal-opportunity disease. It doesn't stop when your circumstances change. As long as you plan ahead, however, those circumstances need not pose insurmountable problems. In this chapter you'll learn how to cope with diabetes when you're pregnant, need dental work, or are caring for a diabetic who's very young or very old.

DIABETES AND PREGNANCY

Diabetes was once considered an absolute prohibition against pregnancy. In the nineteen thirties fetal mortality in pregnant diabetic women was forty-five percent. That figure has declined steadily in the decades since then, to today's averages of two to four percent. What's made the difference? Once again it's blood-glucose control. It seems that poor blood-sugar control is what has the greatest impact on fetal survival.

If you're a diabetic woman who's planning pregnancy, it's crucial to get your condition under control first. Well-managed diabetes is no longer thought to pose any special risks during pregnancy, as long as the mother remains under close observation during her term. Indeed, you may not become pregnant at all without good diabetic control: poorly controlled diabetes may interfere with ovulation, resulting in decreased fertility. It's also been associated with an increased risk of extrauterine implantation (implantation of the fertilized egg outside the uterus), or difficulty in estimating the baby's gestational age. What's more, many women are pregnant for two months or more before they realize they're expecting—and it's during those first eight weeks that the infant's developing organ systems are most vulnerable to injury in a less-than-optimal environment. Potential problems among babies born to diabetic women include:

- prematurity

- abnormally large size (macrosomia)

- respiratory problems

- heart, spine, or skeletal malformations

- low blood calcium

- jaundice

- infections

- difficult birth

These conditions are becoming increasingly rare as doctors learn more about the management of pregnant diabetic women, but good diabetic control before pregnancy is essential.

Ideally, management is a team approach, involving the obstetrician/gynecologist, a pediatrician, and a diabetologist (a doctor who specializes in the treatment of people with diabetes), plus the woman's primary-care physician. The goals of treatment include maintenance of blood glucose at healthy, consistent levels; the achievement of a normal pattern of weight gain (and sufficient weight gain); and the avoidance of metabolic abnormalities like ketosis or hypoglycemia. Pregnancy does not seem to initiate eye or kidney problems in women who did not have these complications before, but it may hasten their progress if the mother had them already. Another goal of therapy, then, is to minimize these complications as much as possible when they exist.

Once your pregnancy is confirmed, you'll probably undergo the following steps:

- a thorough evaluation of your health

- an ultrasound test, which determines the exact age of the fetus

- a test for something called alpha fetoprotein, which is conducted when you're sixteen weeks pregnant to screen for spinal defects in the fetus

- assessment of your blood-glucose control at least once every trimester

- an eye examination and an electrocardiogram (ECG), which helps determine the condition of your blood vessels and heart

- regular monitoring of your kidney function

In addition it's critical that you continue your SMBG, perhaps doing it even more often than you did before. This is the best tool you have to assess the status of your diabetic control. It might even be a good idea to review your SMBG procedure with your doctor, nurse, or diabetes educator, just to be safe. The hormonal and metabolic changes that occur during pregnancy usually cause your blood-sugar levels to change, and frequent SMBG will help you and your health-care team decide upon appropriate adjustments in your insulin dose as your pregnancy proceeds.

For the first trimester most diabetic women don't need any changes in their insulin regime, but some women become hypoglycemic and must reduce the dose. Hormonal changes during the second and third trimester may lead to insulin resistance, meaning you'll have to increase your dose to maintain a safe blood-sugar level. By the end of their pregnancies many diabetic women find that they're taking insulin at two or three times their prepregnancy levels, especially since doctors often set new, lower target blood-glucose levels to strive for when pregnant. That's because maternal blood glucose dips during pregnancy, even in women who are not diabetic.*

In addition to SMBG, regular urine tests for ketones are also critical when you're pregnant. At high enough levels these substances can cross the placenta and enter the baby's circulation, where they may affect the developing brain; even worse, they may kill the fetus. This is still another reason why good glucose control is so important during pregnancy.

If you want to assure yourself the best prenatal care, find

* Insulin does not cross the placenta, so it cannot enter the baby's circulation, and is therefore safe to use during pregnancy.

an obstetrician who's affiliated with a hospital that treats large numbers of pregnant, diabetic women. That may increase your chances of a successful pregnancy.

The Other Patient

Today most obstetricians say they treat two patients: the mother and the baby. Along with regular checkups of your health your doctor will probably monitor your developing baby's health as well. In particular he'll most likely watch for normal growth and head development as well as check fetal heartbeat and fetal movements. All of this can be done with special equipment designed to give doctors a picture of the baby's development in the uterus.

Changes in Diet

It's important to gain enough weight when you're expecting, but don't use pregnancy as a license to pig out! This isn't a good idea for any woman, but it's especially risky for the diabetic, who has to keep strict tabs on her blood sugar. The two to four pounds you'll probably gain during your first trimester won't require any changes in diet. During your second trimester your nutritionist will probably have you add two hundred calories a day, and another hundred calories a day in the third trimester. Most doctors today consider twenty-five to thirty pounds to be a safe total weight gain during pregnancy.

Gestational Diabetes Mellitus (GDM)

Some nondiabetic women develop diabetes during the second half of their pregnancies. This condition, called gestational diabetes mellitus (GDM), is most likely in women with one or more of these characteristics:

- pregnancy past age thirty-five

- GDM during one or more previous pregnancies

- a previous pregnancy resulting in a baby with a birth weight of more than nine and a half pounds

- a family history of diabetes

- other symptoms of diabetes or high levels of glucose in the urine

It is not always possible to predict who will develop GDM, so the American Diabetes Association recommends that all pregnant nondiabetic women be screened for it at twenty-four to twenty-eight weeks of pregnancy. Women with GDM usually have no obvious symptoms and don't require special treatment, except a carefully planned diet and exercise routine to keep their blood glucose within normal range. A woman whose blood glucose shoots extremely high may need temporary treatment with insulin.

GDM usually subsides after delivery, but the women who develop it have a greater risk of developing diabetes some months or years following the pregnancy, especially if their babies weigh more than nine pounds at birth.

JUVENILE DIABETES:
SOME TIPS FOR PARENTS

Few situations in life are more agonizing than having a child with a chronic disease, especially one that requires the child to take daily shots and pay careful attention to his food and exercise. Other siblings may resent the extra time parents must give a diabetic child, and people outside the family may respond with prejudice or even cruelty. Susie, a ten-year-old who's had diabetes since she was three, recently came home from school in tears. "The other kids tease me because I have to take medicine," she told her mother. "Then, at recess, they wave candy bars in my face and laugh at me because I can't have them." Susie's parents finally had to send her to a private school, but it wasn't because of the other children. She had a mild hypoglycemic episode during class and had to take some emergency glucose she'd brought with her. The school later contacted Susie's parents and told them that, as a "handicapped" child, she'd have to attend a special school. No one in the public school was "authorized" to give Susie glucose if she couldn't do it herself, so they couldn't take the responsibility of teaching a diabetic child.

At least Susie was old enough to talk to. A diabetic infant cannot tell his parents how he feels. Babies cry in response to a variety of stimuli—how can parents distinguish hypoglycemic irritability from ordinary hunger, or distress over a dirty diaper? Toddlers may talk to you, but as anyone who's ever cared for a two-year-old will confirm, the word they most often say is *no*. Temper tantrums may prevent you from recognizing symptoms of hypo- or hyperglycemia, from giving injections, or performing blood tests. Anxious parents may, on the other hand, sometimes confuse a child's tantrum or moodiness with hypoglycemia. It's not hard to see why parents caring for very young children with diabetes often report feeling lonely and overwhelmed.

As they approach school age, children can be taught to do their own SMBG and to recognize the symptoms of hypoglycemia. They can participate in meal planning and may even learn to give themselves injections. Nevertheless they still require constant supervision, since an unexpected game of tag or a few bites of a classmate's cookie may wreak havoc on blood-sugar levels.

Some tips to remember when raising a diabetic child:

1. Increase his responsibility for self-care as he gets older. A child who actively participates in his own treatment is more likely to take that care seriously. Also, the more knowledgeable he is about his care, the better equipped he'll be to handle emergencies and special situations.

2. Try not to let one child's diabetes disrupt the entire family. Be alert to signs of excessive tension or hostility, especially on the part of siblings who may be jealous of the extra attention a diabetic child needs. Seek counseling if necessary.

3. When your child starts school, make sure school personnel know what to do for a diabetic child in an emergency. Alert them that hypoglycemia may produce unexpected changes in thinking and behavior. Fortunately, most school employees are more enlightened than those Susie's family encountered.

4. The American Diabetes Association and the Juvenile Diabetes Foundation have many books and pamphlets about childhood diabetes—some written for parents,

others for the young patients themselves. In addition they have information about local support groups that may help you cope when some of the feelings may become too much. Consult your local chapter or the national headquarters of the ADA or JDF; you'll find the information in the last chapter.

The Diabetic Adolescent

Puberty is stormy enough without the special claims of diabetes. The teenager's desire for independence and control is directly at odds with a condition that demands careful planning of meals, medication, and activity. So it's not surprising that many teens don't adhere to their schedules for eating or taking their shots and may ignore injunctions against spontaneous activity—an impromptu bike ride, for example—without the right precautions. Some doctors find that they must negotiate for certain levels of cooperation. For example, a teen who resists performing frequent SMBG may agree to test his urine once a day. Clearly this compromise should be used in only the most stubborn patients, but as a last resort it's better than nothing.

Some adolescents engage in bizarre behavior, like decreasing their insulin shots in an effort to lose weight; a shy teen may exaggerate the disease's demands to avoid socializing or taking risks.

For all of these reasons and more, adolescents respond best when the benefits of their treatment are made obvious and when instructions are simple and clear, and preferably written down. For example, a teen who balks at following his diet, taking insulin, or testing his blood or urine may be more cooperative if parents associate those tasks directly with his ability to drive or participate in sports. However, parents and health-care providers should allow as much flexibility as possible on issues like diet and exercise. A teenager may become resentful if doctor's appointments disrupt other activities, if he has to travel a long way to see the doctor, and if he's kept waiting in the office. If he wishes, an adolescent may see the doctor alone, with the understanding that the doctor will tell the parents about the results of the visit, but only in front of the patient himself.

A teenager who experiences frequent episodes of DKA is probably not adhering to his treatment program and may require counseling if the episodes persist.

DIABETES IN THE ELDERLY

At the opposite end of the spectrum elderly diabetics may not adhere to their regimen, but for entirely different reasons. Problems with vision or manual dexterity may interfere with handling syringes or glucose meters, while hearing or memory loss may keep these patients from following instructions properly. Kidney function also declines with age, putting the elderly at greater risk of diabetic kidney complications. Finally, physical limitations combined with emotional changes like depression or feelings of isolation may interfere with eating on schedule or reduce the motivation for self-care in general.

This does not, of course, apply to every elderly patient. Many people, diabetics included, remain healthy and vigorous to the end of their lives. But for someone on whom age has taken a greater toll, the following tips may help:

1. If the patient's mental capacity is diminished, keep the regimen simple. Avoid complicated instructions or algorithms in favor of a routine that merely concentrates on avoiding hypo- or hyperglycemia.

2. Preserve normal routine as much as possible. Keep changes to a minimum.

3. Have the doctor perform glycosylated hemoglobin tests several times a year to monitor the patient's blood-glucose control.

4. Meal plans should also be kept simple. Aim for balanced meals that account for the patient's habits and tastes. If you're caring for an elderly diabetic, make sure she's eating enough. Insufficient food intake is a problem for many older people.

5. Make foot care a priority. If it's too hard for you to see or reach your feet, ask someone to check them for you and schedule regular visits to a podiatrist. If you're caring for someone with diabetes, see to it that her feet are regularly checked, by you, the patient, or a health-care professional.

6. The diabetic should have a thorough checkup, including the eyes and feet, at least every three months. Make sure any instructions are written down in simple language.

7. Elderly patients who live alone and have trouble getting around or preparing meals may wish to take advantage of community services such as the Visiting Nurse Association or Meals on Wheels. Your local chapter of the American Diabetes Association can give you more information about these and other organizations.

SURGERY IN THE DIABETIC PATIENT

In general the risks of surgery don't seem to be any greater for the diabetic than they are for anyone else. The one exception is emergency surgery, which does not permit enough time to evaluate and prepare the patient. If you have diabetes, many experts recommend that you wear a "dog tag" or carry a card stating that fact, so in case of an accident or emergency your caretakers can allow for your special needs.

A diabetologist should be part of the health-care team of any diabetic who's planning to undergo surgery. Your primary-care physician should know, of course, about any surgery you're going to have. He'll undoubtedly want to evaluate your condition thoroughly, paying special attention to any complications, especially those of the kidney or heart. Surgery in the diabetic does require some special precautions by your medical team, so it's best to find a surgeon and an anesthesiologist experienced in the treatment of people with diabetes.

DIABETES AND DENTAL CARE

As with surgery, dental care in a well-controlled diabetic need not be any more complicated than it is for nondiabetics. There's some controversy over the likelihood of periodontal (gum) disease; while some experts think diabetics run a greater risk, others claim that periodontal disease has no special affinity for diabetics, but once it appears in the diabetic, it progresses more quickly than it would in someone else. And, as with every other complication, the poorer the diabetic control, the worse the periodontal disease.

Other dental manifestations of uncontrolled diabetes include:

- delayed wound healing

- poor response to infection

Sometimes:

- dry mouth

- inflammation of lips or tongue

- early tooth loss

- fungal infections of the mouth

Periodontal disease usually starts when oral bacteria accumulate and cause a condition known as gingivitis, or inflammation of the gums. Gum bleeding in response to pressure, as when you brush your teeth or when a dentist probes, is the most obvious symptom of gingivitis. Periodontal disease occurs when the gingivitis extends to the bone. In advanced cases periodontitis may lead to bone loss and require surgery for treatment.

The factor initiating both these conditions is bacterial accumulation, and anything that impairs your body's ability to fight these bacteria will increase your risk of periodontal disease. Diabetes, which affects immune-system function, is one such factor. Hence the increased severity of gingivitis and periodontitis in diabetics.

The best way to avoid these problems is through the practice of good dental hygiene. Along with daily brushing, flossing is important because most periodontal problems occur between the teeth, where a toothbrush can't reach.

In their early stages a thorough cleaning by a dental hygien-
ist may be all that's necessary to reverse gingivitis or periodontitis. Later stages of these conditions, however, will
require deeper cleaning or possibly even surgery.

Oral surgery is no riskier for the well-controlled diabetic
than it is for anyone else, but you do have to plan ahead and
take some precautions. If possible it's best to receive local
anesthesia, because that won't interfere with your ability to
take your insulin and to have meals or snacks. You'll probably be instructed to avoid food for at least six hours before
surgery, so it's best to schedule the operation for the early
morning so the only meal you'll miss will be breakfast. Diabetic patients often receive an intravenous glucose infusion
during surgery, which should provide them with the same
amount of carbohydrate they would have gotten in the meal
they missed. In addition you may be told to take half your
insulin dose before the operation and the other half after.

Don't neglect good dental hygiene once things are back
to normal. If you don't brush and floss your teeth every day
and get regular dental checkups, the bacteria will simply
return, and the problems will start all over again.

Tips for Diabetic Dental Care

1. Use a soft-bristled brush on your teeth and floss every
   night before bed. It's also a good idea to massage your
   gums gently, using a finger or the little rubber imple-
   ment on the end of many toothbrushes.

2. Get dental checkups every two to three months.

3. Make sure your dentist has your primary physician's phone number. It's sometimes important for the two to consult each other; your dentist should inform your doctor if he treats you for an oral infection, since this may affect your blood-glucose level and your insulin dose.

4. To diminish the risk of hypoglycemia, schedule dental appointments for the morning, after breakfast, whenever possible. Try to arrange things so that you're not subjected to a long wait in the office, as this can disrupt your meal/medication schedule. Take your usual morning insulin dose before seeing the dentist.

5. You must get adequate nutrition even if the dental work leaves you unable to eat. Ask your dietitian to plan a few meals consisting of soft or liquid foods, in anticipation of such an event.

6. Some kinds of dental procedures may injure your gums and leave you at risk of infection, especially if you have a heart murmur or find it difficult to control your blood glucose. Ask your doctor if he thinks you should take antibiotics in conjunction with your dental work as a precaution.

7. Trauma or stress may raise your blood-sugar level. Keep dental appointments short; if you need extensive work, have it done over the course of several visits.

EIGHT

WHERE TO FIND MORE INFORMATION

Diabetes research is extensive, and expanding as we move into the twenty-first century. More and more public funds are being allotted for experiments as scientists discover better treatments for this disease and its complications. A diabetes cure remains elusive, but if one is possible, it's just a matter of time before researchers find it.

Diabetics are fortunate in one respect: because of all this funding and research there's a large network of support and information available. Virtually all of it is free, or at least affordable within most budgets. Because diabetes affects so many organ systems, most of the major medical organizations in this country have some information about diabetes as it relates to their particular specialty. In addition there are two organizations devoted entirely to diabetes, and the vast resources of the National Institutes of Health are also available.

What follows is a list of organizations that can help you find information on almost any diabetes-related subject you can imagine. If the organization doesn't have the information itself, it can direct you to a person or place that does. Many of these societies can also tell you about local physicians, support groups, and diabetes information classes. Don't be afraid to ask questions and request information. Remember: You can't be overeducated when it comes to your health.

American Diabetes Association
National Service Center
1660 Duke Street
Alexandria, VA 22314
(800) 232-3472

This private, voluntary organization fosters public awareness of diabetes and supports and promotes diabetes research. It has printed information on many aspects of diabetes, and local affiliates sponsor community programs. In addition it offers memberships for a nominal sum to diabetics and other people interested in diabetes; as a member you receive a monthly magazine that discusses the latest developments in diabetes care, nutrition, and exercise. You'll also find interviews with prominent diabetics, who discuss how they handle their disease.

The ADA has local chapters in most large cities; if your community has one, it will be listed in the phone book. Or you can call the number given above and ask for more information.

American Dietetic Association
216 West Jackson Boulevard
Suite 800
Chicago, IL 60606
(312) 899-0040

This professional society of dietitians and nutritionists can help you locate a diet counselor in your community. It also provides a form of quality control by allowing qualified applicants to register with the association; these individuals can then call themselves registered dietitians, or RDs. Having an RD means a dietitian has completed an approved course of study and served as an intern in a clinic or hospital. You should get your nutritional advice *only* from someone with an RD.

American Heart Association
7320 Greenville Avenue
Dallas, TX 75231
(214) 373-6300

The AHA is a private, voluntary organization that has information on heart disease and how to prevent it. Most major cities have local AHA affiliates; consult your phone book.

Juvenile Diabetes Foundation International
432 Park Avenue South
New York, NY 10016
(212) 889-7575

A private, voluntary organization for people interested in Type I (juvenile onset) diabetes. As with the ADA and AHA, the JDF has local affiliates around the country. Check your phone book or contact them at the number above.

National Diabetes Information Clearinghouse
National Institute of Diabetes and Digestive
and Kidney Diseases
Box NDIC
Bethesda, MD 20892
(301) 496-3583

Affiliated with the National Institutes of Health, the publicly funded NDIC offers a wealth of information on many aspects of diabetes, for free or at nominal cost. Call or write and ask for a list of their publications and recommended books. They may also be able to give you information about diabetes organizations or support groups in your community.

National Eye Institute
Building 31, Room 6A32
National Institutes of Health
9000 Rockville Pike
Bethesda, MD 20892
(301) 496-5248

Another component of the National Institutes of Health, the National Eye Institute offers information on eye disease and diabetes.

National Heart, Lung, and Blood Institute
Building 31, Room 4A21
National Institutes of Health
9000 Rockville Pike
Bethesda, MD 20892
(301) 496-4236

The NHLBI offers information on heart disease, for which diabetics are at higher-than-average risk.

GLOSSARY

This glossary contains words that have appeared in the text that may be new to you. It also contains words that may not have appeared in this book, but that you may encounter as you do more reading on the subject of diabetes.

A

adipose tissue: The scientific term for the fat tissue, the tissue in which the body's fat stores occur.

adrenaline: A hormone, also called epinephrine, that is secreted by the adrenal glands, which sit on top of the kidneys. Often called the "fight or flight" hormone, adrenaline helps the liver release glucose and limits the secretion of insulin from the pancreas. This hormone also makes the heart beat faster and raises blood pressure.

aldose reductase inhibitors: A group of drugs that shows promise in the treatment of certain diabetic complications, such as neuropathy.

algorithm: A plan developed by your doctor telling you what changes in food, exercise, or medication to make if circumstances that affect your blood sugar change.

amino acid: A component of protein. A protein molecule is made up of long chains of amino acids strung together; insulin is one such protein. When you eat protein, the digestive tract breaks it down into its amino acids, which are absorbed into the bloodstream and, in nondiabetics, elicit the secretion of insulin.

arteriosclerosis: Hardening of the arteries. Atherosclerosis is one form of arteriosclerosis. People with diabetes are at higher-than-average risk of developing this condition.

atherosclerosis: A form of arteriosclerosis characterized by the buildup of plaque (defined below), which is thought to be related to factors such as high blood cholesterol, high blood levels of certain fats, cigarette smoking, high blood pressure, and diabetes.

autonomic neuropathy: A complication of diabetes resulting in damage to the nerves that govern involuntary actions such as digestion.

B

background retinopathy: A complication of diabetes resulting in damage to the small blood vessels in the retina, the light-sensitive tissue lining the back of the eye. Background retinopathy is an early form of eye damage and, if caught and treated in time, causes few if any symptoms.

basal infusion: A slow, steady trickle of insulin released into the bloodstream by an insulin pump.

bolus infusion: In diabetics using an insulin pump, an extra burst of insulin that the patient releases at times of special need, such as after a meal.

C

carbohydrate: One of the three main sources of energy for the body. Carbohydrates are mainly sugars and starches that the body breaks down into glucose. The body also uses carbohydrates to make a substance called glycogen, that the liver and muscles store for future use. Without enough insulin the body cannot use carbohydrates properly, resulting in diabetes.

cataract: A lens of the eye that has become clouded over, due to age or disease. Diabetics seem to be at higher risk of developing cataracts.

complex carbohydrate: Commonly known as starch, complex carbohydrates are substances composed of hundreds of carbohydrate molecules. During digestion they are broken down into their simpler carbohydrate components and absorbed into the bloodstream, where they raise blood sugar and, in nondiabetics, elicit the secretion of insulin from the pancreas.

D

diabetes mellitus: The condition that results when the pancreas cannot make insulin, or when the insulin is defective or the body is resistant to it in some way. Untreated diabetes is characterized by extremely high blood sugar, excessive hunger, thirst, and urination, and eventually a coma and death.

diabetic ketoacidosis (DKA): The condition that results when a diabetic's body must burn fat instead of carbohydrate to obtain the energy it needs. This process causes the formation of substances known as ketones. High levels of ketones in the blood distort the blood's acid-base balance, which eventually disrupts brain function, which may lead to a coma and, if not corrected, death.

diabetologist: A physician who specializes in the treatment of people with diabetes.

E

epinephrine: See **adrenaline,** above.

F

fiber: The indigestible form of carbohydrate found in most vegetables and fruits. Although it's not digested, fiber helps to maintain regularity and may help regulate blood sugar. There's also evidence that fiber helps keep blood cholesterol low and helps prevent certain forms of cancer.

fructose: A type of sugar found in many fruits and vegetables, and in honey. Fructose is often used as a sweetener in "diabetic" foods because, unlike glucose, it does not require insulin to enter the cells.

G

gestational diabetes mellitus (GDM): A type of diabetes that occurs in some nondiabetic women during the second half of their pregnancies. In most cases blood-glucose levels return to normal after delivery, but these women do run a higher risk of developing diabetes some months or years following the pregnancy.

gingivitis: An inflammation of the gums that, if left untreated, may progress to serious periodontal disease.

glucagon: A hormone released by the pancreas whose action is the opposite of that of insulin: it raises the level of glucose in the blood.

glucose: A simple sugar found in the blood. It is the body's main source of energy. Glucose is sometimes called dextrose.

glucose tolerance: The term sometimes used to refer to the body's utilization of glucose. Diabetics are said to have impaired glucose tolerance.

glycemic index: The effect certain foods seem to have on raising or lowering blood sugar. Diabetics are sometimes told to select foods, usually starches, with a lower glycemic index, but many experts now question its reliability in predicting blood-sugar changes and do not recommend its use.

glycogen: The form in which the liver and muscles store carbohydrate. Glycogen consists of simple carbohydrate molecules linked together in a chain. When blood sugar dips too low, these organs can break the chain to use the carbohydrate molecules for fuel, or send them into the bloodstream to raise blood sugar.

glycosylated hemoglobin test: A blood test performed by a doctor in which he measures the amount of glucose attached to the patient's hemoglobin. From this the doctor gets an idea of the patient's average blood-glucose levels over the past four to eight weeks.

gram: A small unit of measurement, equal to approximately one thirtieth of an ounce.

H

hemoglobin AIC: The form of hemoglobin measured in a glycosylated hemoglobin test.

honeymoon phase: A phase of renewed insulin production by the pancreas that sometimes occurs when newly diagnosed Type I diabetics, particularly teenagers and young adults, are placed on insulin therapy. During the honeymoon phase the patient's need for insulin therapy may diminish drastically; some patients may be able to eliminate their shots altogether. The honeymoon phase may last for up to a year, but it is temporary and the patient will eventually have to resume taking insulin.

hyperglycemia: The condition of excessively high blood sugar, usually greater than 140 mg/dl (fasting) or 200 mg/dl (after a meal). Hyperglycemia is the hallmark of untreated diabetes.

hyperlipidemia: The condition of having too much fat in the blood. Hyperlipidemia is associated with an increased risk of heart disease.

hypertension: The medical term for high blood pressure, which occurs when the blood flows through the arteries with greater-than-normal force. This condition strains the heart, harms the arteries, and increases the risk of stroke, heart attack, or kidney problems.

hypoglycemia: The condition of excessively low blood sugar, usually less than 50 to 60 mg/dl.

I

impaired glucose tolerance: The condition that results from diabetes. Glucose tolerance is considered impaired when the glucose that enters the body from a meal cannot enter the cells, usually because of deficient or faulty insulin production. Hyperglycemia results from impaired glucose tolerance.

insoluble fiber: The form of fiber found in wheat bran and other whole grains. Insoluble fiber helps speed the passage of food through the digestive tract.

insulin: The hormone whose faulty or deficient production leads to the development of diabetes. Insulin allows glucose and amino acids to enter organs such as muscles, which then use the glucose for fuel. Without insulin, glucose cannot enter these organs and builds up in the bloodstream; this may ultimately cause all sorts of complications. Without glucose the organs cannot function properly and resort to the same emergency metabolic measures they would use if the body were truly starving. This exacerbates the symptoms and complications seen in diabetes.

insulin-dependent diabetes mellitus (IDDM): Also called juvenile-onset or Type 1 diabetes, this form of the disease is characterized by onset before age twenty and the body's complete loss of the ability to produce insulin.

insulin pump: A device that delivers a constant trickle of insulin into the bloodstream through a catheter inserted under the skin. Insulin pumps can also deliver a burst, or bolus, of insulin, whenever it's needed, such as just before meals.

insulin resistance: The condition that results when the body's tissues can no longer respond to the insulin that's produced. This may be due to some flaw in the insulin itself, a loss of special insulin receptor sites on the tissue, or a combination of both.

J

juvenile-onset diabetes (JOD): See **insulin-dependent diabetes mellitus,** above.

K

kernicterus: A disorder that sometimes occurs in the central nervous system of a developing fetus. The results may be deafness, seizures, or cerebral palsy. The incidence of kernicterus seems higher in the babies of diabetic women who were not well controlled during pregnancy.

ketoacidosis: The condition that results when the body uses fat as its primary source of fuel. Fat metabolism results in waste products called ketones. If ketones accumulate in the blood, as they might in untreated diabetes, they alter the body's acid-base balance and interfere with brain function. If not treated promptly, ketoacidosis may result in death.

ketosis: See **ketoacidosis,** above.

kilogram: A unit of measurement referring to one thousand grams, or about two and one-fifth pounds.

M

macrosomia: Abnormally large size of a newborn baby, sometimes seen in children born to women with diabetes.

macula: The central portion of the retina of the eye, responsible for precise vision like that needed for reading or driving.

macular edema: A condition that develops when blood vessels in the macula leak fluid or blood into macular tissue, causing it to swell. This may result in serious vision impairment. Macular edema is one possible form of diabetic retinal damage.

maturity-onset diabetes (MOD): Also called Type II or noninsulin-dependent diabetes mellitus (NIDDM), this form of diabetes usually, but not always, occurs in obese people over the age of forty. These patients may still make some insulin, but either their tissues do not respond to it (insulin resistance) or the insulin is defective in some way. Most diabetics—some ninety percent—have this form of the disease.

milligram: One thousandth of a gram.

N

nephropathy: The medical term for kidney damage.

neuropathy: The medical term for nerve damage. There are two major forms of diabetic neuropathy: autonomic neuropathy and peripheral neuropathy.

noninsulin-dependent diabetes mellitus (NIDDM): See **maturity-onset diabetes (MOD),** opposite.

O

obesity: The condition of being at least twenty percent above one's ideal body weight.

ophthalmologist: A doctor who specializes in treating diseases of the eye.

oral hypoglycemics: Drugs used to treat some people with Type II diabetes. In the United States today oral hypoglycemics all belong to a group of compounds known as sulfonylureas.

orthostatic hypotension: An abrupt drop in blood pressure that may occur upon standing suddenly, which leads to feelings of dizziness or lightheadedness. In diabetics, orthostatic hypotension is sometimes a symptom of autonomic neuropathy.

P

periodontal disease: An advanced form of gum inflammation that extends to the bone and may require surgery. Periodontal disease seems to occur with greater severity in diabetics.

peripheral neuropathy: A form of diabetic nerve damage affecting the nerves serving the arms, legs, hands, and feet. The feet are at particular risk of injury due to peripheral neuropathy.

plaque: 1. The substances that build up in certain major arteries, thought to consist of cholesterol, fat, chemicals in cigarette smoke, and other items. Extensive plaque may block the arteries that carry blood to nourish the heart muscle; when this happens a heart attack may result. 2. The buildup of metabolic substances produced by bacteria on teeth. These substances are thought to be involved in the development of tooth decay or gingivitis.

podiatrist: A practitioner specializing in treating diseases of the feet.

postprandial: Following a meal.

proliferative retinopathy: The proliferation of small, fragile blood vessels in the retina, which may then break and bleed into the eye, often with serious consequences to vision. Proliferative retinopathy is one potential complication of diabetes.

R

retina: The light-sensitive tissue that lines the back of the eye and helps transmit visual signals to the brain.

S

simple carbohydrate: Another word for sugar. Blood glucose is a form of simple carbohydrate. When connected together in a long chain, simple carbohydrates form complex carbohydrate, or starch.

soluble fiber: The form of fiber found in oat bran and fruits and vegetables. Some people think soluble fiber in the diet helps regulate blood glucose, but other experts have challenged this assertion.

sucrose: Another word for table sugar. Sucrose consists of two simple carbohydrates, glucose and fructose, linked together.

sugar: See **simple carbohydrate,** above.

sulfonylureas: See **oral hypoglycemics,** above.

U

uremia: Blood poisoning that results when the kidneys cannot filter waste products out of the blood.

V

vitrectomy: Removal of the vitreous humor, the gellike substance found in the eye.

INDEX

ABOUT THE AUTHOR

Norra Tannenhaus holds degrees in biopsychology and nutrition from Vassar College and Columbia University. She has written extensively on health, medicine, and nutrition for consumers and publications, and her magazine articles have appeared in such major publications as *Self, Glamour,* and *Mademoiselle*. She is the author of *Learning to Live with Chronic IBS*. *What You Can Do About Diabetes* is her fifth book. A New Yorker at heart, Norra Tannenhaus currently makes her home in Los Angeles.